# Culture and Knowledge

Edited by Friedrich G. Wallner

Vol. 17

PETER LANG

Frankfurt am Main · Berlin · Bern · Bruxelles · New York · Oxford · Wien

Friedrich G. Wallner
Fengli Lan
Martin J. Jandl
(eds.)

# Chinese Medicine and Intercultural Philosophy

## Theory, Methodology and Structure of Chinese Medicine

PETER LANG
Internationaler Verlag der Wissenschaften

**Bibliographic Information published by the Deutsche Nationalbibliothek**
The Deutsche Nationalbibliothek lists this publication in the Deutsche Nationalbibliografie; detailed bibliographic data is available in the internet at http://dnb.d-nb.de.

Cover illustration:
"Nike von Samothraki"
Courtesy of Kovac-Verlag.

Supported by the Austrian Ministry
of Science and Research, the Cultural Department
of the Municipal of Vienna and Robert Rogner jr.

ISSN 1613-902X
ISBN 978-3-631-60556-1


Internationaler Verlag der Wissenschaften
Frankfurt am Main 2011


www.peterlang.de

# Table of Contents

Friedrich G. Wallner

# Chinese Medicine: A Challenge for Philosophy of Science

In this lecture I will discuss the issue: Why does Chinese medicine challenge philosophy of science? At the first glance it seems to be possible to hold a view for which this issue is not crucial, namely the position that Chinese medicine and philosophy of science have no point in common, i.e. to state that Chinese medicine and philosophy of science stem from two totally different realms that are not and cannot be connected. However, I hold the opposite view: If philosophy of science fails to explain the specific structural principles of the proposition system called Chinese medicine, than Chinese medicine will perish. The failure of philosophy of science will destroy the proposition system that is now (and formerly) known as Chinese medicine; perhaps a proposition system will survive the failure of philosophy of science that will bear the name of Chinese medicine – but it won't be the Chinese medicine we know since many centuries.

This lecture is subdivided into two parts: Firstly, I discuss the intellectual commotions caused by two important books in philosophy of science and the consequences I draw of the poor situation of philosophy of science at the end of the 1980ies; secondly, I will depict how Chinese medicine could be reflected, and I will present my own research strategy that deals correctly with what is know as cultural relativism – I will emphasize the self-understanding of Chinese medicine as Qu Xiang Bi Lei.

## 1. Philosophy of science and the development of Constructive Realism

In the last 50 years philosophy of science developed in a strange, but nonetheless interesting way. There were phases characterised by a high likelihood that philosophy of science will lose its right to exist. Philosophy of science, it should not be forgotten, is a very young discipline. It emerges as autonomous discipline in the field of philosophy between Ernst Mach and the Vienna Circle, and it is due to the Vienna Circle philosophers having established philosophy of science. That was about 100 years ago, and since about 50 years philosophy of science has been critically ill.

The reason for its being ill is simply to be found. Thomas Kuhn published his famous book on the structure of scientific revolutions that clearly shows that the history of science should not be interpreted as a history of progress, but as a history of total change in certain periods. The change from the Ptolemaic physics to the Copernican physics was a change of the view point that cannot be explained as intellectual development. The progress of science does not exist, but a change of paradigms, and this change is socially driven.

Kuhn met mostly with ignorance. It was alleged that Kuhn simply did not understand what philosophy of science is about. The most famous proponent of this camp is – easily to guess – Sir Karl Popper who holds that Kuhn speaks about facts of intellectual history, but he himself speaks about norms in scientific research. This division performed by Popper is a typical outcome of the European argumentation way: There are two worlds – the world of facts and the world of norms or ideals. Popper was deeply convinced that he did not touch facts, but that he actually touched norms. I am not willing to comment this view here; but I argued hard with Popper in this point.

About 10 years later another book upset the community of philosophers of science, namely “Against Method” by Paul Feyerabend. Feyerabend was familiar with the Vienna Circle philosophy, a scholar of Wittgenstein and Popper, and he actually demonstrates that philosophy of science does not critically analyses science – as it was the outspoken ideal of the beginning days of the Vienna circle –, but that philosophy of science uncritically upholds the scientificy of science. It is a delight to study Feyerabend's analysis, and it is also a delight to read the replies of his colleagues. I remember a number of colleagues who actually declared Feyerabend to be batty. But it is not the place and time to hold forth about this issue here.

There are numbers of interpretations of Feyerabend's views, and it is not always clear which interpretation is correct; sometimes it was even not clear how Feyerabend himself wanted to be understood. Some philosophers – perhaps the majority – see in Feyerabend a destructive philosopher. This behaviour is often to be found, and we will meet it in the behaviour of non Chinese people against Chinese medicine. This behaviour is the exclusion of views by application of the killer phrase that the view of the proponent is not scientific.

Another behaviour was caused by Feyerabend's impressive book – resignation. This resignation results from Feyerabend's insight that primarily social processes reign over science – what, then, has a philosopher of science to do? Not the intellectual analysis is important, but sociological analysis. There seems to be no place for intellectually speaking about knowledge claim of science.

But let's turn to the positive effects of Feyerabend's book. In the first place we can state a new interest for other cultures. This cultural turn shows the way out of the crises. By the way, Richard Rorty formulates in "The Mirror of Nature" views that are similar to mine, but in the "Mirror" there is this strange fiction in the starting passage.

At this point, my own philosophy of science comes into the play. At the time when Feyerabend's book was published, I was concerned with analysis of science, especially of physics. After the works of Kuhn and Feyerabend philosophy of science has lost his authority to tell scientists what they have to do. Nevertheless, my colleagues either resigned or did exactly this – they explained to scientists what they actually do. I voted for a third alternative by performing a turn: I asked scientists what they need from philosophy. I developed an interest in the interests of scientists in philosophy. At this point I realised that philosophy of science since its beginning was nothing else than metaphysical speculation, i.e. there was no real contact to scientists. After my turn the work with scientists clearly showed: Scientists are able to applicate adequate methods, but they do not understand what this application means for the world or for truth. It is due to Aristotle to have seen that humans do not only want to have things functioning, but that humans also want to understand why things work. And scientists utter exactly this point – they do not only want to be able to applicate their methods, but they want to gain insights that go beyond the mere handling of data. In short, scientists want to understand their constructs in the context of their culture.

And here is an important claim of Constructive Realism, the philosophy of science that I developed as an answer to the situation of philosophy of science in the late 1980ies: Science yields knowledge if science is able to outline cultural convictions sharply and clearly. Constructive Realism is built on the insight that philosophy of science has not to fulfil the task of seeking failures in the argumentations of scientists, i.e. by applying logical formulas or by analysing test arrangements. This kind of critics is concerned with the instrumentalist aspect of science. What should be at the core of philosophical analysis are the cultural prerequisites of theories (and methods).

2. The situation of Chinese medicine and why it needs an adequate philosophy of science

Nowadays there is no universally valid understanding of what Chinese medicine is. Just consider the wide spread term TCM or Traditional Chinese Medicine. It must be stated that Chinese medicine is not to be equated with TCM since TCM is an artificial construct built on some, but clearly not on all classical texts of Chinese medicine. The famous sinologist Paul Unschuld uses to say that TCM is made by the central committee of the Chinese Communist party. This view is slightly exaggerated, but it is true that in 1956 under the surveillance of the central committee a specific set of texts were declared to be the main TCM corpus. TCM then was offered to the rest of the world. In other words: TCM does not mirror what Chinese medicine actually and in the full sense is.

What are the main differences between TCM and Chinese medicine? TCM is "pragmatist", i.e. TCM is success oriented and influenced by scientific materialism and communism. But, on the other hand, in its original version Chinese medicine is connected with a set of Chinese arts and sciences and is a form of an interdisciplinary art. A crucial point for the understanding of Chinese medicine reads: The body and the human is an effigy of the world. And then there is the special view of subjectivity in Chinese medicine. We Europeans cannot understand that the well known distinction between object and subject is a relatively new invention of Western philosophy. And we should expect that we cannot find this differentiation in a medicine that is some thousand years old. And hence in Chinese medicine subjectivity is very important, but subjectivity should not be misunderstood in the modern philosophical sense. Subjectivity in Chinese medicine means the emotional and intellectual touch of the patient. The Chinese physician is not an expert, but healing is a process between two people. Chinese medicine, genuinely practised, is not objective! (Here: "objective" in the Western sense.)

Constructive Realism offers the means to understand science as cultural construct. That scientific systems depend on culture is one of the most important constructive-realistic claims. Because of this cultural basis of scientific systems it is possible to claim without contradiction that contrary scientific systems are all true. Even if two scientific systems – say Western medicine and Chinese medicine – are contradictory, we will state that both are true – that's a very important argumentation strategy of Constructive Realism. What is necessary to claim that this argumentation strategy is not batty? We just have to take into account that every claim for truth is based on a cultural prerequisite and that no scientific system escapes its cultural fundament. Hence the important insight of Constructive Realism reads: There is no unconditioned truth. Truth is relational concept. Truth is not absolute, i.e. detached from its cultural breeding ground (so to speak).

But how is it possible to handle different claims for truth? How to deal with sciences if we take their cultural basis for serious? In order to answer this question I developed a method that is similar to hermeneutics, i.e. strangification. Strangification means to take a proposition system out of its framework and to put it into the framework of another culture. The first "success" of this displacement is probably confusion. In the first moment you are not able to understand what happens. Therefore you ask where the confusion comes from. At this moment you see that the confusion results from different background information scientists have for using a language. The confusion resulting from strangification is due to the fact that language use in science is only possible if you follow a lot of rules which are not explicitly formulated. Strangification, thus, gives insight into rules another science is implicitly working with.

A further issue to be discussed here is the difference in the medical practices of Chinese and Western medicine. There is no mysticism in the medical practice of Chinese medicine, that's not the difference. Rather both medicines differ in the manner of reference: In Western medicine medical practice refers to theories, in Chinese medicine medical practice refers to paradigms. The Western doctor orders symptoms according to a theory expressed in universal laws, the Chinese doctor assigns symptoms to paradigms that are samples of collected experience. Therefore in Chinese medicine there are formulations about the "heat" or the "cold" in the body that often sound funny in the ears of a Western doctor. The Western doctor takes the patient's temperature (i.e. he measures the heat), the Chinese doctor uses heat as ordering paradigm. Chinese heat can't be measured by means of Western medicine, to do so results from a misunderstanding of Chinese medicine.

By the way, a crucial difference between Western and Chinese thinking concerns the Western ascription of every event to something material. The background of this way of thinking is the historical emancipation of science vis-à-vis the Catholic Church. In this process the material and causal explanation was overemphasized. Chinese thinking is very different: function and relation are core ideas.

But I must drop a remark to what is known as culture relativism. Culture relativism overemphasizes culture to a reason of action and thinking: Because someone is European or Chinese etc., he has to act in a European or Chinese way. In this way we find a typical European motive in the foundation of intercultural relationships. Even if Europe wants to take other cultures serious, it cannot jump over its own shadow. According to this culture-relativist view culture is an ordering instance. It commands what and how to think and to act.

By application of the strangification method I found many structural features of Chinese medicine and of Chinese thinking, but also of Western medicine. Just imagine the following strangification: We ask: What is reality in Chinese thinking and what is reality in Western thinking? The analysis shows that the views are incompatible. The classical European idea reads: What does not change, that is real. The realm of reality is characterised by changelessness and constancy. The next step in European intellectual history is that this claim of changelessness is connected with truth –constancy only is the fundament of truth. In a sharp contrast, Chinese people do not relate to things, but to phenomena. And I made an interesting observation: Chinese people are not interested in the truth, unchangeable background of phenomena. No, Chinese people and philosophers stop their consideration at the level of phenomena. And, believe me, nothing lacks! The question what there is behind phenomena is absurd in Chinese thinking.

Western science goes behind phenomena; Chinese science does not have the faintest idea of this analysis level. Chinese science opts for another way of explanation. Phenomena are seen in their intercorrelations and in their relation to human action. This methodological analysis level conforms to the aim of Chinese science: The aim is to control the succession of phenomena. Changes are always seen in connection. The central method of Chinese science is called Qu Xiang Bi Lei; it connects phenomena based on structural features.

My strangifications between Western and Chinese science showed that there is an important difference in ontology. In the Western world the universe is grasped as constructed, in China the universe is conceived as interwoven, i.e. everything is connected with everything and the whole universe. Therefore I suggest that system theory is adequate for the reflection on Chinese culture and Chinese medicine, because system theory is a Western theory that emphasizes the mutual connectedness of events and facts.

Fengli Lan

# Intercultural Philosophy and Chinese Medicine: Reflections of Philosophy of Chinese Medicine in Chinese Language

Abstract: Chinese philosophy and science (including Chinese medicine) presupposes Chinese Culture. Chinese classical philosophy focuses on the study of "Tao", probing into the "Tao of the Universe" and the "Tao of Man" from various angles. Philosophy of Chinese medicine is an important component part of Chinese classical philosophy, and also an original philosophy of science originated from Chinese culture, which produces Chinese classical science. The author reflects philosophy of Chinese medicine in Chinese language from its ontology, methodology, ultimate aim, and epistemology, and concludes that Chinese medicine can be correctly and fully understood in the network of intercultural philosophy.

## Introduction

The word "philosophy" is of Greek origin "φιλοσοφία, *philosophía*", composed of "philien (love)" and "sophia (wisdom)", and so originally means "to love wisdom". Philosophy is defined as "the rational investigation of the truths and principles of being, knowledge, or conduct".[1] Chinese translation of "philosophy" is 哲学 (zhe xue), and came into Chinese vocabulary about 100 years ago via translation. But Chinese philosophy evolved from the remote antiquity (the late period of patrilineal clan commune 唐虞时代) and formed in the Shang-Zhou dynasties (C.1600-221B.C.), so has at least over 3000 years of history. Chinese classical philosophy, in brief, focuses on the study of "Tao", probing into the "Tao of the Universe" and the "Tao of Man" from various angles.

Philosophy is in principle a product of a specific culture (including a specific cultural need and cultural convictions based on philosophy), and this statement is valid for all forms of philosophy, including European philosophy and Chinese philosophy. Pointedly speaking, European philoso-

1 Webster's Encyclopaedic Unabridged Dictionary of the English Language (New Revised Edition) [Z]. New York: Gramercy Books, 1994: 1082.

phy and science (science emerges from philosophy, historically seen) presupposes necessarily European culture; while Chinese philosophy and science presupposes Chinese Culture.[1]

I support the viewpoint that the philosophy, science, and medicine are pluralistic just like the cultures are diverse. China has her own unique culture, philosophy, science, and medicine, which are very different from that of the West. Chinese medicine, the only live form and also the representative of Chinese classical sciences, no doubt presupposes Chinese philosophy and Chinese culture. The author first discusses cultural connotations of philosophy of Chinese medicine, and then reflects philosophy of Chinese medicine in Chinese language from its ontology, methodology, ultimate aim, and epistemology, and finally concludes that Chinese medicine can be correctly and fully understood in the network of intercultural philosophy.

## 1. Cultural Connotations of Philosophy of Chinese Medicine

Philosophy of Chinese medicine is an important component part of Chinese philosophy, and also an original philosophy of science from Chinese culture.

### 1.1 Philosophy of Chinese Medicine: An Important Component Part of Chinese Philosophy

Chinese medicine emerges and develops in the soil of Chinese classical culture, of which Chinese philosophy is the core, and so in essence Chinese medicine presupposes Chinese philosophy. It can be easily seen from that Qi, Yin-Yang, and five phases, the major concepts of the philosophical structure of Chinese medicine, all underwent the evolution from philosophy to medicine through metaphorizing.[2]

---

1 Wallner, Friedrich G. Intercultural Philosophy: The Viennese Program. Wallner, Schmidsberger, & Wimmer (eds). Intercultural Philosophy: Aspects and Methods, Frankfurt am Main, 2010: 13-20.

2 Note: Metaphorizing: *Qu-xiang Bi-lei* is the methodology to form metaphors of Chinese medicine, therefore I propose that *Qu-xiang Bi-lei* is the metaphorizing process of metaphors of Chinese medicine. See the paper: Lan Fengli. Metaphorizing: the Way to Bridge *The Book of Changes* and Chinese Medicine. In Wallner, Schmidsberger, & Wimmer (eds). Intercultural Philosophy: Aspects and Methods, Frankfurt am Main, 2010: 177-192.

Actually, philosophy of Chinese medicine is in essence the same as Chinese philosophy, in specific, is mainly the application of the philosophy of *The Book of Changes*, of Taoism in the field of Chinese medicine, which demonstrates the great significance of cultural and philosophical dependency of Chinese medicine. Philosophically speaking, *The Book of Changes*, *Lao Tzu*, and *Huang Di's Inner Classic* present with the systematic intimate relationship with Tao as the focus: *The Book of Changes* lays the philosophical foundation for Tao of all kinds; *Lao Tzu* proposes that Tao abides by the nature; and *Huang Di's Inner Classic* advocates that medicine abides by Tao, i.e. the nature.

1.1.1 *Tian Ren He Yi:* the Philosophical Foundation for Tao of All Kinds

The theme of Chinese philosophy is to probe into the relationship between the "universe and man", or the relationship between "the Way of Universe and the Way of Man", regarding the Universe as Man's Universe and Man as Universe's Man.[1]

*The Book of Changes* establishes *Tian Ren He Yi* 天人合一 or the Universe and Man uniting and resembling each other by making a far-fetched comparison between them. It states that "In the remote antiquity, the way that Fu Xi 伏羲 ruled the country was that raising his head to observe the images of the heaven, bowing his head to observe the principles of the earth, observing the similarities between the patterns of birds and beasts and those of mountains on the earth, taking near images from man and taking far images from the universe (to compare them so as to understand them). Then he started to make the Eight Trigrams (ba gua, 八卦) in order to understand the integrity of the divinities and to analogize myriads of beings in the universe", which lays the philosophical foundation for Tao of all kinds in Chinese culture and medicine, which formed through metaphorizing.

Here the formation of the Tao of Chinese medicine is the case in point. So, how the Tao of Chinese medicine formed? Or what is the relationship between *The Book of Changes* and Chinese medicine – one deals with *Xiang Shu* (images and numbers, 象数) and their implicit mean-

---

1 Note: *Tian* in *Tian* Tao and *Ren* Tao *or Tian Ren He Yi* is usually translated into Heaven, but not the same as in the West, the better translation is Universe.

ings in the universe, while the other talks about health and illnesses of man? Actually they are talking about the same thing in essence by applying metaphors or metaphorizing: life – one on the life of the cosmos and the other on the life of man. Both are open systems, both are communicated with and related to each other, and both should be in a state of harmony in itself and with the other, otherwise problems or illnesses will ensue, which is radically different from the strict divisions between the life and the inanimate, the subject and the object, the man and the nature etc. in the Western culture. Maybe it is fantastic for the Westerners that *The Book of Changes* and Chinese medicine do not reduce life or being to something material like cells, proteins, genes, etc., instead they understand life or being by establishing and interpreting something symbolic like *gua* 卦 and *yao* 爻, Qi, yin and yang, the eight trigrams, the five phases, the images and numbers, the visceral image, and so on.[1]

It's worth to note that most of the thinking ways of Chinese medicine originate from *The Book of Changes* and are established through metaphorizing. ① The Thinking Way of *Xiang Shu* (images and numbers, 象数 ): The *Zang Xiang* (Visceral Image, 藏象) theory is established on the basis of elementary understanding of the organs to explain physiological functions of man through *Qu-Xiang Bi-Lei* (taking image and reasoning from analogy, 取象比类); and "pattern identification and treatment" is set up by summarizing and generalizing various symptoms and signs into a certain "pattern image" also through *Qu-Xiang Bi-Lei.* ② The Thinking Way of *Bian Yi* (changing, 变易): Chinese medicine regards life, health and illnesses as constantly changing processes, and stresses not only the transmission and transformation of illnesses, but also institutes corresponding treatments to meet the changes. ③ The Thinking Way of Holistic Approach: *The Book of Changes* establishes *Tian Ren He Yi* 天人合一 or the Universe and Man Uniting and Resembling each other, on the basis of which the theoretical system of Chinese medicine has formed. Chinese medicine regards man as an organic whole, and also studies the physiology and pathology of man in the unity and mutual relations of man, nature and society, thereby administers corresponding healthcare methods.

---

1 Lan Fengli. Metaphorizing: the Way to Bridge *The Book of Changes* and Chinese Medicine. In Wallner, Schmidsberger, & Wimmer (eds). Intercultural Philosophy: Aspects and Methods. Frankfurt am Main, 2010: 177-192.

To sum up, *Tian Ren He Yi* is the philosophical foundation for Tao of all kinds in Chinese culture and science. Here medicine is the case in point. Metaphorizing is the way to bridge the thinking ways and metaphors of *The Book of Changes* and Chinese medicine such as "—" and "- -" and yin-yang, the eight trigrams and the five phases, the five phases and the visceral image, etc.[1], and the way to establish the Tao of Chinese medicine.

1.1.2 Tao 道: The Way of the Nature and Medicine

*Huang Di's Inner Classic* is the highest authority on philosophy of Chinese medicine, and also one of the most important classics on Taoism of Chinese philosophy.[2] Taoism focuses on the study of "Tao", and *Lao Tzu* and *Chuang Tzu* are the most important classics of Taoism.

Tao 道 was originally written as " 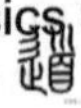 ", following the part of "辵", which actually shows an image of a man walking on a way with his eyes big open, metaphorizing "the only way you must follow or take in order to go ahead" . Its original meaning is explained in *The Origin of Chinese Characters* as "the way to walk", which indicates the direction for the walker, is the route to a certain destination, and then is metapharized to mean law, rule, or principle. Besides, Tao 道 in the ancient times had several other extended meanings: thinking system or theory such as in *The Analects• Living in brotherliness* (*Lun Yu • Li Ren* 论语•里仁) "My thinking system is run through by a central idea"; to govern or manage explained in *Guang Ya • Shi Gu* (广雅 •释诂); way or method such as in *The Book of Shang Yang's Ideas* (商君书•更法) "There is not just one way to govern the society". Also, the character 道 resembles the shape of 首 head, thereby bearing the meaning of start or beginning. You see that Tao 道 bears so many meanings, therefore, as a fundamental philosophical concept; its connotations are deep, subtle and complicated.

It is *Lao Tzu* that discusses Tao as an abstract concept and endows it with a philosophical meaning of "embracing all". *Lao Tzu· Chapter 25*

---

1 Lan Fengli. Metaphorizing: the Way to Bridge *The Book of Changes* and Chinese Medicine. In Wallner, Schmidsberger, & Wimmer (eds). Intercultural Philosophy: Aspects and Methods, Frankfurt am Main, 2010: 177-192.

2 Ni, Maoshing. The Yellow Emperor's Classic of Medicine [M]. Boston, Massachusetts: Shambhala, 1995: Back-Cover.

states that "Therefore, Tao is great. Heaven is great. Earth is great. Man is great. In the universe, there are four great things, and man is one of them. Man abides by the earth. Earth abides by the heaven. Heaven abides by Tao. Tao abides by the nature"; The Chapter 42 states that "Tao begets One (Qi). One begets Two (Yin-Yang). Two begets Three (the integration of Yin and Yang). Three begets all things. All things carry Yin and embrace Yang, where the central and harmonious Qi makes them in harmony", which shows the generation of all things in the universe from Tao (*Wu* 无 or Nothing) to all things (*You* 有 or existence). That is to say, Tao is the origin of all things in the universe and the Way which must be observed by all.

In Chinese medicine, *Huang Di's Inner Classic* states that "Yin and yang are the Tao or Way of the heaven and earth, the fundamental principles of the myriad things, the origin of all changes and transformations, the root of generating and killing, the palace of man's spirit" in *Plain Questions• Images Corresponding to Yin-Yang* (素问·阴阳应象大论).[1] It also states that "Of all things in between the heaven and earth, nothing is more precious than man.

Man lives on the Qi in between the heaven and earth, and grows in accordance with the law of the seasons" in *Plain Questions• Discourse on Protecting Life and Preserving Physical Appearance* (素问·宝命全形论). *The Origin of Chinese Characters·Man Part* (说文解字·人部) also states that "Man is the most valuable being in between the heaven and earth".

Thereby, it can be seen from the above quotations that "Heaven", "Earth", and "Man" are independent from and closely related to each other, and they compose a whole system, in which man plays the leading role; and that the thinking way of the "heaven-earth-man" in *Lao Tzu* embodies the thinking way of the universe, which is specified in the *Inner Classic* as the thinking way of the Chinese medicine, which shows that the great progress of natural philosophy in the aspect of the nature replacing the God. In *Lao Tzu*, Tao abides by the nature; In the *Inner Classic*, medicine abides by the Tao; In essence, medicine abides by the nature. Holistic ap-

1 Note: The translations of the quotations from *Huang Di Nei Jing Su Wen* all accord with Guo Aichun's interpretation in his book *Textual Criticisms, Annotations, Modern Language Interpretation of Huang Di Nei Jing Su Wen* (2nd Ed.), published by Tianjin Science and Technology Press (Tianjin, China) in 1999.

proach and individualized treatment based on pattern identification with the aim for the central and harmonious state in health care and disease treatment are all embodied in *Lao Tzu* and *the Inner Classic.*

*Chuang Tzu* carries on *Lao Tzu*'s Tao of the nature, and advocates that man was born in between the heaven and earth, and so should follow the way of the nature, i.e. the way of Yin-Yang and the seasons, in health care. It also states the way of cultivating the spirit - "to do nothing that is left undone" and "to be indifferent to any fame or gain". These ideas are all embodied in the *Inner Classic.*[1] Therefore, Tao abides by the nature, and medicine abides by Tao, and so medicine abides by the nature, which is the Tao of Chinese medicine.

### 1.2 Philosophy of Chinese Medicine: An Original Philosophy of Science Originated from Chinese Culture

There is a major misunderstanding that Chinese philosophy mainly discusses society, politics, and ethics, but neglects the nature. Actually, agriculture, astronomy, geography, mathematics, and medicine of the ancient China were very advanced, and even more advanced than that of the West esp. before 14th century. That is to say, Chinese philosophy of the nature and life in probing into the relationship between the Universe and Man produced all of the Chinese traditional natural sciences, which worked very well before or even has worked quite well until today. For example, Du Jiang Yan 都江堰, the water control and irrigation dam, which has been listed in the World Inheritance Name List and was designed and built in accordance with the classical scientific ideas, has been working so well in preventing serious flooding for over 2000 years, and even survives the Sichuan Earthquake in 2008; While cracks appeared in a modern big dam made of concrete mixer after the earthquake in 2008, which was designed and built nowadays according to the modern science. So, it's clear that Chinese classical sciences have their own unique values.

Today, only Chinese medicine survives ever after facing the serious challenges from Western medicine, and almost all of the other Chinese classical natural sciences like agriculture, astronomy, geography, and

---

1 See the chapters of *Tian Shi* 天适 and *Ke Yi* 刻意 of *Chuang Tzu* 庄子, and the chapter *On the Prenatal True Qi of the Remote Antiquity* of *Plain Questions* 素问・上古天真论 for more details.

mathematics etc. have declined and are totally replaced by the corresponding Western natural sciences. It is a great pity. But the fact also indicates philosophy of Chinese science fits much better with the living system than with the other systems, and the living system is the only one which is always in a state of constant changing and transforming.

Undoubtedly, Chinese medicine works quite well in treating many illnesses, which usually cannot be successfully treated by Western medicine. That's why Chinese medicine arouses so great interests in studying Chinese medicine among researchers of different fields of study both at home and abroad. Generally speaking, most of them try to find out the scientific evidence on mechanism of Chinese medicine mainly by doing lab experiments and clinical trials (such as RCT) as the same way in researching Western medicine, but few of them research Chinese medicine in its philosophical foundation. The point is that the outcome of your research will be doubtful or will not go along with nor enrich the theoretical system of Chinese medicine if you do not understand its philosophical background.

There is a common Chinese misinterpretation of philosophy of Chinese medicine, which is extensively written into the textbooks of Chinese medicine for higher education of China. That is, Chinese medicine is established on the rudimentary materialism and dialects, which actually results from understanding Chinese medicine with the framework of Western philosophy. Thereby, some scholars believe that Chinese medicine still lingers in the stage of pre-science or infancy of modern science, and advance that Chinese medicine must get rid of its philosophical concepts like Qi, yin-yang, five phases if it needs to be modernized and scientific. Actually, it's totally wrong. Chinese medicine will definitely lose its strong points if it is modernized and studied in this way.

Chinese medicine must be scientific for it has worked so well in prevention and treatment of so many illnesses for thousands of years. The point is that Chinese medicine is closer to humanities not science in the common Western sense, and it's based on an original philosophy of science originated from Chinese culture.

Then, how to define philosophy of Chinese medicine? It is a kind of original philosophy of science originated from Chinese culture with the focus on *Xiang* 象 (phenomena and images) and relationships. It stresses phenomena, images, and functions more than morphological structures, stresses relationships among the beings esp. among the live man, the nature and the society more than causality (whys), stresses integration more than separation, stresses the constant changes and transformations more than unchanged features, and stresses perceptual understanding more than quantified measurement, etc. So philosophy of Chinese medicine is not at all rudimentary materialism for materialism will definitely lead to reductionism; and yin-yang theory emphasizes phenomena and images (such as the images corresponding to yin-yang 阴阳应象) and dynamic harmony in a whole system, while dichotomy stresses separation and opposition, and so philosophy of Chinese medicine is not at all rudimentary dialectics.

What philosophy of Chinese medicine mainly deals with is the Tao, Qi-Yin-Yang-Five Phases, thinking way, methodology, perspectives on life, disease, and treatment of Chinese medicine, which are applied to construct the theoretical system of Chinese medicine, to expound the physiology (normal state, ping 平) and pathology (diseased states, bing 病) of man, and to guide diagnosis and treatment of illnesses. Thereby, philosophy and medical knowledge, i.e. the basic correct understanding of the body, health and illnesses are integrated into an organic whole, i.e. Chinese medicine, a unique medical system originated from Chinese culture. So, we can say that Chinese medicine is the product of the integration of science (medical knowledge) and culture (its philosophical foundation), bearing both cultural and scientific connotations.

Why do the majors of Chinese medicine always go back to the Four Great Classics of 2000 years ago? That is to say, why is there no breakthrough but only development and enrichment since the establishment of the knowledge system? Why has Chinese medicine not been developing along the similar procedure to Western medicine? The answer is that the philosophy of Chinese medicine makes the system of Chinese medicine into a self-contained and fruitful paradigm, which can be enriched and developed in the same framework – *Qu-Xiang Bi-Lei* guided by *Tian Ren He Yi* established at that time, and survive up till today. You can get clearer idea from the following Table.

Table 1 *Different Views of Heart in Hippocratic Corpus and Huang Di Nei Jing*

| **Heart** | ***Hippocratic Corpus*** | ***Huang Di Nei Jing*** |
|---|---|---|
| **General Understanding** | Two atriums and two ventricles; | The organ as a Monarch, from which spirit originates; the root of life, the seat of the spirit; the greater yang within yang; |
| **Main Functions** | The right atrium provides lungs with blood, accepts air from lungs, exchanges air; | Rules the body's blood and vessels; opens into the tongue; it's brilliance manifests in the face; |
| **Relations to Others** | There is only air, no blood in the left atrium;<br>the left atrium is the location of intrinsic heat. | South, summer, hot & fire, bitter, red, zheng, elation, laughing, and the Heart, etc. all correspond to fire in the five elemental phases; the heart (fire) engenders the spleen (earth). |
| **Outcome** | A Morphological Heart Organ: Focuses on the morphological structure of the heart, thus providing direction, possibilities and leaving space for the further study on its anatomical structure and corresponding physiological functions | A Heart Complex System: Separates "Heart" from the organ "Heart" in anatomical sense, integrates "Heart" with the theories of Yin-Yang and Five Phases, social phenomena (Monarch), natural phenomena (season, direction, climate, flavor, color), and other aspects of man (spirit, joy, tongue, face, spleen) into "A Heart Complex System |
| **Analysis** | Guides Western medicine to develop on the philosophical foundation of reductionism, mechanism and dichotomy, thus embodying the analytical thinking | Establishes the theory of Visceral Image (**藏象学说**), embodying the holistic approach "Four Seasons - Five Zang Organs – Yin-Yang" and "Universe and Man Uniting and Resembling Each Other" |
| **Conclusion** | Western Medicine continuously refreshes itself because of the application of advanced scientific technology and instruments (tools) | Chinese Medicine has formed a self-contained fruitful paradigm, so can be enriched and developed in the same framework - *Qu-Xiang Bi-Lei* guided by *Tian Ren He Yi* established about 2000 years ago, survive up till today. |

Note: Here the contents from *Hippocratic Corpus* are translated into English from the Chinese translation.

## 2. Reflections of Philosophy of Chinese Medicine in Chinese Language

Language is the outcome of the culture. (Claude Levi Strauss) Language is redefined as "*the means and process of man cognizing, understanding and stating the world*".[1] The founding of philosophy of language at the beginning of the last century is another "Copernican revolution" in the history of philosophy,[2] which has deeply influenced the philosophy of science, highlighting the vital role of linguistic analysis in the scientific methodology, thus promoting the development of modern logic. Modern logic stresses the role of language, regards a scientific theory as a language system, being composed of word items, sentences, and their logic relationships.

### 2.1 Ideographic Writing and Philosophy of Chinese Medicine

Chinese characters are the only ideographic writing (as opposed to phonetic writing) which has been preserved for over 5,000 years in the world. The shape of a Chinese character is directly related to its meaning, and both integrate into a unity. The formation of a Chinese character, an organic whole of the shape and the meaning, is one-step made following the rule of the nature, reflecting the direct communication between and unification of the subject and the object. The formation also implies an important methodology, i.e. *Qu-Xiang Bi-Lei* 取象比类.[3] Now the author takes *Qi* 气, *Xiang* 象, and *He* 和 to illustrate the ontology, the methodology, and the ultimate aim of philosophy of Chinese medicine.

#### 2.1.1 *Qi* 气 Explains Ontology of Philosophy of Chinese Medicine

Chinese philosophy applies the concept of *Qi* to explain the nature of existence. *The Origin of Chinese Characters • Qi Part* （说文解字•气部）

---

1 Pan Wenguo. Redefining Language: Means and Process of Man Cognizing and Stating the Genuine World [J]. (Hongkong) Chinese Philology Correspondence. 2002, 2: 33-36.

2 Xu Youyu. "Copernican" Revolution: Linguistic Transfer in Philosophy [M]. Shanghai: Joint Publishing House, 1994: 1.

3 Lan Fengli. Globalization of TCM: Differences between TCM and Western Medicine. In Wallner, Lan & Jandl (eds.).The Way of Thinking: Theory, Methodology and Structure of Chinese Medicine [C]. Frunkfurt am Main: Peter Lang, 2010: 24-44.

states that "*Qi* refers to thin, floating clouds. The character 气 [1] is an ideographic character." The character 气 in *Jia Gu Wen* 甲骨文, the inscriptions on bones or tortoise shells of the Shang Dynasty (c. $16^{th}$-$11^{th}$ century B.C.), was written as "川", which resembles air current, evaporating and rising, whose image is just like cloud, will disappear very soon and become invisible. Therefore, *Qi* is invisible and formless, exists everywhere, can be gathered into a form, for instance, *Qi* can be condensed into water.

Soon afterwards, the *Qi* which surrounds and congests the Man's space was abstracted into the *Qi* which bears a philosophical sense. Philosophers of the Spring Autumn and Warring States Periods (770-221B.C.) believed that *Qi* is the basic ingredient constituting the world, and also the basic ingredient constituting the Man and that everything in the universe comes into being by the movement and mutation of *Qi*, as stated in *The Book of Changes* "everything is transformed and generated by the enshrouding [Qi] of the heaven and earth".

*The Book of Changes* establishes *Tian Ren He Yi* 天人合一 or the Universe and Man Uniting and Resembling Each Other by making a far-fetched comparison between them. *Tian Ren He Yi* actually indicates that the Universe and the Man constitute in the same way, i.e. being composed of the same ingredient – *Qi* in the same order. Therefore, *Qi* becomes the foundation of *Tian Ren He Yi*.

Later on, ancient Chinese medical experts introduced "*Qi*" into the medical field at the right moment. In the time of *Huangdi's Inner Classic*, "*Qi*" is regarded not only as the basic ingredient constituting the world, but also as the basic ingredient constituting the Man which can be transformed into blood, essence, and body fluid, etc., and the normal functional activities of the life which is governed by "*Qi*" is known as *Shen* or spirit.

According to *A Concise Dictionary of Chinese Medicine* (简明中医词典),[2] *Qi* in Chinese medicine bears the following meanings: ① nutritious, essential substance flowing inside the body, such as food qi, breathed air. ② functional activities of the *zang-fu* organs in a general sense, such as

1 The character 氣 is not the original form of 气 but a mistake during the evolution of Chinese characters, which means "feed and grain for the guests" according to *The Origin of Chinese Characters • Rice Part.*

2 Li Jingwei, Qu Yongxin, Yu Ying'ao, et al. A Concise Dictionary of Chinese Medicine. Beijing: China Press of Traditional Chinese Medicine, 2001: 173.

visceral *Qi* (i.e, the functional activities of the *zang-fu* organs); *Qi* can also be classified into original *Qi*, nutritive *Qi*, defensive *Qi*, *pectoral Qi*, etc. according to its source, distribution, and function. ③ the location or stage of pattern identification of warm diseases.

That is to say, *Qi* in philosophy of Chinese medicine is to make man become man, and the logic function implied in the *Wei* (Defense) – *Qi* – *Ying* (Construction) – Blood Pattern Identification for treatment of warm diseases is the condition of processes and activities of life, i.e. *Qi* is the condition for what it is conditioned, which is similar to Plato's ideas. Plato's ideas are the conditions of the understanding of things and of the beings of the things. Some conceptual aspects of *Qi* have the same argumentative function as Plato's theory of ideas.[1]

Be aware, ancient Chinese philosophy regards *Qi* as the ontology of the universe, and stresses *Qi*'s material characteristics - the basic ingredient constituting the universe; while in philosophy of Chinese medicine, *Qi* is the unification of material aspect and functional activities – *Qi* is not only the basic ingredient constituting the Man, but is also used to expound the dynamic processes and functional activities of the life.

Here is worth to note that the concept of *Qi* in Chinese culture is radically different from the concept of material in Western culture, a Chinese misinterpretation. *Guan Tzu* （管子） states that "*Qi* can be limitedlessly small and limitedlessly big". Therefore, *Qi*, the origin of the universe and life, is formless without any boundaries or any separation of two opposites (dichotomy). So man can feel *Qi* for man is a being of the integration of the body and the mind, of the subject and the object, of the material and function. The concept of material in the Western culture must be something with a form even with the rapid development of understanding the structure of materials. Materialism is a philosophical foundation of Western natural science, which stresses the separation and opposition of the body and the mind, of the subject and the object, and greatly promotes the development of modern Western science.

It's necessary to know that Yin-Yang, the five phases, and the eight trigrams are all the subdivisions of *Qi* of different levels from the viewpoint of *Qi*, which indicates a gradual generating and evolving process from *Qi*

1 Note: The ideas here are enlightened by personal talks with Prof. Friedrich Wallner.

to Yin-Yang then to the Five Phases then to the Eight Trigrams. *The Book of Changes* (周易) states that "the changes have *taiji* (the Supreme Ultimate, the Absolute in ancient Chinese cosmology, presented as the primary source of all created things, i.e. *Qi*) , *taiji* generates yin and yang, yin and yang generate the four images, i.e. the greater yang, the greater yin, the lesser yang, and the lesser yin, and the four images generate the eight trigrams". That is to say, *Qi* can be transformed into yin and yang, yin and yang can generate and be transformed into the five phases which are composed of two pairs of yin and yang (water and fire, wood and metal) plus one middle soil. Actually, the four images and the eight trigrams indicate the five phases although the term "five phases" does not appear in this quotation: The four images can be regarded as four phases, i.e. water, fire, wood, and metal; the eight trigrams can be regarded as water (yin), fire (yang), wood (yin wood and yang wood), metal (yin metal and yang metal), and soil (yin soil and yang soil).

Therefore, the formless *Qi* explains the ontology of philosophy of Chinese medicine, i.e., in the structure of Chinese philosophy, *Qi* has the corresponding place of the Western ontology, and is also the foundation of the model of *Qi*, Yin-Yang, and the Five Phases.

### 2.1.2 *Xiang* 象 Implies Methodology of Philosophy of Chinese Medicine[1]

*Xiang* 象, one of the most important metaphors of Chinese culture, runs through almost every aspect of Chinese culture like philosophy, medicine, ideographic writing, arts and other sciences. Then, what is meant by *xiang*? The original meaning of "*xiang*" as stated in *The Origin of Chinese Characters* （说文解字）"*xiang*, with long nose and teeth, is a big mammal in the Southern *Yue* area", refers to elephant. In remote antiquity, the elephant had lived in the Central Plains of China. Later on, the elephant had to migrate south because of the changes in climate, so the people in the Central Plains had few opportunities to see elephant again. Han Fei Zi （韩非子）, a famous philosopher and the representative of the Legalists of the late Warring States Period (475-221B.C.), said in his *Jie Lao Pian* (解老篇) that "people seldom see the live elephant, but has gained the

1 Lan Fengli. Metaphor, *Qu-xiang Bi-lei* and Chinese Medicine. In Wallner, Lan & Jandl (eds.). The Way of Chinese Thinking: Theory, Methodology and Structure of Chinese Medicine. Frankfurt am Main: Peter Lang, 2010: 63-88.

skeleton of a dead one, so they can imagine what it is like after investigating the picture or image of its skeleton. Therefore, all in people's imagination is known as '*xiang*'". This quotation also reveals the mystery of the origin of the Chinese compound "xiang xiang" (想象, literally "thinking or imagining elephant", means imagination), setting off "xiang 象"'s "imagining" cultural connotations.

In the meanwhile, we can see that "*xiang*" originally evolved from "seeking similarities" between things from the angle of genetics, which is also stated in *The Book of Changes*: "*xiang* refers to something being alike or resembling this thing". Transforming *xiang* into a cultural symbol is related to divining activities - *Bu* 卜 with tortoise shell and *shi* 筮 with stalk of *shi* grass – the two main ways to hunt for information of the cosmos in the Yin-Zhou dynasties (C1600-256B.C.). *Zuo's Spring and Autumn Annals ·the Fifteenth Year of Xi Gong's Reign* （左传·僖公十五年） states that "tortoise is *xiang*"; *The Book of Changes* states that "change is *xiang*". That is to say, the omens on the tortoise shell and the trigrams were called *xiang* for they were regarded as being capable of communicating the *Tian* 天 with the Man and ruling all of the cultural information. Thereafter, *xiang* has become a symbol which carries all the cultural information. In Chinese traditional culture, all of the sceneries, the sun, the moon, the stars, even Man's pulses, tongues and viscera are termed together with *xiang* like jing (scenery) *xiang*, ri (sun) *xiang*, yue (moon) *xiang*, xing (star) *xiang*, mai (pulse) *xiang*, she (tongue) *xiang* and zang (visceral) *xiang*; Tao, the primitive motive force of the origin of everything in the universe, is also known as *xiang,* the big *xiang* (大象).

*Xiang* implies a vital methodology of philosophy of Chinese medicine: *Qu-xiang Bi-lei* 取象比类 or taking image and reasoning from analogy, which can be summarized into four steps as stated in *The Book of Changes*: 1) Observing object or phenomenon (*guan wu* 观物): directly observing an object or phenomenon; 2)Taking image (*qu xiang* 取象): summarizing and refining the *image* of the object or phenomenon after repeatedly observing and feeling it; 3) Comparing and analogizing (*bi lei* 比类): comparing the things which need to know with the "*image* (*xiang* 象)"; 4) Understanding the Way or Rule (*ti dao* 体道): finding the rules. *Qu-xiang Bi-lei* results in the formation of metaphors, and such metaphors show the process of *Qu-xiang Bi-lei* and the relationship of the involved things or objects or phenomena or images.

*Qu-xiang Bi-lei* is the core methodology of philosophy of Chinese medicine to know the cosmos and man, to construct and develop the theoretical system and clinical explorations of Chinese medicine. We can say that Chinese culture is *Xiang* culture, and Chinese science is *Xiang* Science, and Chinese medicine is a *Xiang* medicine, which stresses relationships among beings in the universe.

2.1.3 *He* 和 Shows Ultimate Aim of Philosophy of Chinese Medicine

"*He* 和" is usually translated into "harmony" in the Western world, which shows a simplified and reduced understanding of this concept by the Westerners. This concept as shown by its original form bears two aspects of meaning: the first is different, the second is harmonious. That is to say, being both different and harmonious can be termed "*He* 和".

It is really indeed the case that the simplified Chinese characters (the popular style of writing now in China) have also reduced the cultural connotations implied in their original forms. 和 is the simplified form of the character 龢. As stated in *The Origin of Chinese Characters* ( 说文解字 ), its original form is composed of two parts: the left part is an ideographic part symbolizing a musical instrument made of bamboo with three holes used to harmonize different tones, and the right part 禾 is phonetic part, indicating its pronunciation He; Its original meaning refers to harmony of different music tones.

The development of Chinese characters show that harmony of different foods is known as 鬹 (the upper part means to harmonize, the lower part 甘, means sweet, which is applied to harmonize the other tastes i.e. sour, bitter, pungent and salty. See *The Origin of Chinese Characters*·甘 *part,* 说文解字•甘部), harmony of different medicinal herbs is known as 藥 (medicine), harmony of different tones is known as 樂 (music), one of the variant forms of the character 療 (treat) also has the 樂 part, which shows that restoring harmony is the goal of all the Chinese medical treatments.

It is well known that Chinese medicine uses mixtures of different medicinal substances formulated according to a certain strategy in a holistic approach to disease, i.e. *Yao* (Medicine, 藥), which is different from *Ben Cao* (Materia Medica, 本草). *Ben Cao*, the materia medica, refers to all of the individual medicinal substances with healing properties, i.e. the medicinal substances or the medicinals, including herbs, minerals and animal parts. While *Yao,* 藥, its original Chinese character, is explained to be “harmony of different medicinal substances”, and is used to “treat illnesses” (the character is 疒 with 樂 inside it, a variant form of 療, the simplified character is 疗), i.e. restoring the harmonious state to the individual. Thus, it is clear that *Yao* 藥 refers to the medicine ready to be taken for treating illnesses, which is composed of more than one medicinal substances formulated according to the strategies of *Jun Chen Zuo Shi* or Chief, Associate, Assistant and Guide medicinals, i.e. formula.

Therefore, *he* 和, the ultimate aim of philosophy of Chinese medicine, is in direct line with Chinese culture, which implies the man in a harmonious state or can be achieved to such a harmonious state by applying *Yao* 藥 or non-medication therapies such as acupuncture, moxibustion, and Chinese massage.

### 2.2 Discourse of Chinese Medicine Reflects Epistemology of Chinese Medicine

Ferid Murad, a Nobel Prize winner in medicine (1998), set up a modern research center on Chinese pharmacology named after his name with the collaboration with Shanghai University of Traditional Chinese Medicine in 2003. At that time, he said he was seeking for a language which is able to give a scientific interpretation for pharmacological and molecule mechanisms of the therapeutic effects of Chinese herbal remedies. Chinese medicine has its own discourse, and so why we need to look for another language to interpret it? Is it possible to find such a kind of language?

Wittgenstein believed that language is a kind of picture, which cannot be proved with facts of the real world. That is to say, we do not need to prove or interpret the logic contained in the discourse of Chinese medicine with the so-called scientific method, what we should do is to regard it as a picture in which the discourse of Chinese medicine describes man’s lifestyle – a harmonious state among man, the nature and the society, how man behaves in the daily life to preserve health, to prevent and treat illnesses, which is like a picture of the life world.

According to Wittgenstein’s idea of philosophy of language – “language games”, Chinese medicine is definitely a kind of language, a language game in respect to man, its healthy state, and its connection with the Universe; Western medicine is another language game in respect to the body and its diseases; and the difference between both is that Chinese medicine does not reduce its language but it enriches it by metaphors.

Therefore it makes sense to say: Chinese medicine is a natural language and Western medicine is a formal language. Here is an importance difference for the theoretical understanding of both: Formal languages must be interpreted for getting sense. Natural languages are interpreting themselves.[1]

It's true that the textual criticism, exegetical studies and annotations of ancient medical classics have always been an important academic field of study in Chinese medicine up till now since the era of the *Huang Di's Inner Classic*,[2] which helps the practitioners of Chinese medicine of the past dynasties understand and develop Chinese medicine in both theoretical and clinical explorations.

Now, let's look at the two paragraphs about the origin of man both from the angle of genetics in Chinese Medicine and Western medicine respectively:

> ① "人生于地，悬命于天，天地合气，命之曰人。人能应四时者，天地为之父母"（素问•宝命全形论）。
>
> Translation: Man is born on the earth, hanging his life to the heaven. The union of *Qi* of Heaven and Earth makes up a man. Man can adapt himself to the seasons for the Heaven and Earth are his parents. (*Plain Questions·Discourse on Protecting Life and Preserving Physical Appearance*)
>
> ② "Man is metazoon, triploblastic, chordale, vertebrate, pentadactyle, mammalian, eutherian, primate… The outlines of each of his principal system of organs may be traced back, like those of other mammals, to the fishes." (L.A.B.-orradaile)
>
> '译文：人属于后生动物，系五趾，三胚层高级动物，属脊索动物门，脊椎动物亚门，哺乳纲，灵长目......象其它哺乳动物一样，他的每一个器官系统的轮廓可以追溯到鱼类。[3]

It is clear that the latter is a kind of formal technical language, a typical language of modern Western science, which is only used as a tool to con-

1 Note: This part is inspired by personal talks with Prof. Friedrich Wallner.

2 Note: For example, the chapter of Zhen Jie of Plain Questions 素问• 针解 and the chapter of Xiao Zhen Jie of the Spirit Pivot 灵枢•小针解 both interpret the chapter of Jiu Zhen Shi Er Yuan of the Spirit Pivot 灵枢 • 九针十二原.

3 Hou Weirui. English Styles of Writing [M]. Shanghai: Shanghai Foreign Language Education Press, 1988: 278.

vey information, to identify its reference, and to express points of view. And it has become so boring and dry by the so-called theoretical and scientific statements. While discourse of Chinese medicine is a kind of hermeneutic language full of metaphors, and it is closely related to the context of the life world – an inseparable organic whole of man, the nature and the society. It can inspire, hint, and enlighten you to know how Chinese medicine understands man in a direct and original way.

According to Wittgenstein's idea of philosophy of language, the discourse of Chinese medicine and that of Western medicine are different "language games", showing different lifestyles, and describing different "pictures" of life, and so one cannot be interpreted or proved by the other. For example, mixing the discourse of Western medicine with that of Chinese medicine will disturb the cognizing way of Chinese medicine, which is just like to coat or cover the transparent life world with the scientific formal language. Therefore, we should reconsider the current progress of researching, modernizing, or even westernizing Chinese medicine, and what we need to do is to understand the rationality of Chinese medicine from its own discourse, from the "picture" of the lifestyle in the life world its discourse describes. That is to interpret Chinese medicine with itself. I do not deny the approach to apply modern science and technology to study Chinese medicine, but such researches must be in accordance with philosophy of Chinese medicine.

## Conclusion

Chinese medicine is an integration of Chinese philosophy and plain understanding of the human life, body and diseases. That is to say, Chinese medicine takes the basic correct understanding of the body, health and illnesses as its prerequisite, *Qi* as its ontological foundation, *Xiang* as its methodological approach, and *He* as its ultimate aim, thereby the Tao of Chinese medicine has formed by following the Tao of the nature under the guidance of *Tian Ren He Yi* or Universe and Man Uniting and Resembling Each Other.

Therefore, it's clear that Chinese medicine presupposes Chinese culture and philosophy; and that philosophy of Chinese medicine cannot be correctly interpreted by Western philosophy, and Chinese medicine cannot be correctly interpreted or proved by Western medicine; and the network of intercultural philosophy provides a correct way to make Chinese medicine fully understandable, can work as a bridge for better mutual understanding of different cultures and different sciences.

*Acknowledgment: I am very grateful to Friedrich Wallner for his inspirations in preparing this manuscript.*

Toru Tani

# The Uniqueness of the World

## Introduction

In this presentation, I would like to clarify some of the methodological problems of research in interculturality *from the viewpoint of phenomenology*. Phenomenological research in interculturality began with *Edmund Husserl*, founder of phenomenology, although it was not a central issue for him. In recent years, various important articles and several full-scale books have been published on this topic. But why is phenomenological and methodological research necessary? Why not simply "compare" cultures. There are many obvious and important cultural differences and, correspondingly, there has been much "comparative" research. But, philosophically speaking, it is also necessary to question the meaning of such "comparisons". Are they truly "purely objective" comparisons[1]? Are comparisons even possible?

The speakers today have been requested by the organizer to "offer the *methodological* problems and results of (our) present research". Methodology is very central for philosophy, but since I believe that every methodology exists in a tense relationship with specific research, I think it is very appropriate that the speakers have also been requested to "discuss their *specific scientific* contribution". But what does "*scientific*" mean here? The notion of "science" relates in some way to "*truth*" and/or "*objectivity*", although all of us here know that it is very difficult to define these notions. The notion of "*culture*" is even more problematic. Because I myself belong to an East-Asian culture, together with some of the other speakers today, I would like to start by examining some East-Asian notions of culture.

---

1 Japanese philosopher, *Tetsuro Watsuji* (1889-1960), discussed the problem of cultural differences in relation to the "wind and earth" (meaning, in this case, "climate" or "environment"). Influenced by Heidegger, he emphasized the openness or "ex-sistere" of human beings to the environment. His argument is highly sophisticated, but his arguments for the "objectivity" of his own description are not sufficient.

There are many cultural differences between different countries in East Asia, which is also the case with Western or European countries. And even within one country, we find distinct differences between different social groups, different generations, and of course, different individuals. Microscopically, there are differences born of every aspect of existence. If this is the case, can we say that a so-called "culture" (such as Japanese culture) really has a solid "unity" or "uniformity"? Probably not. And it seems to me that it is impossible to find a clear distinguishing line *between* cultures: for example, between "Austrian culture", "Japanese culture" and "Chinese culture". All cultures are a "*mixture*" in some sense. And the ratio of mixture is higher today than before. We must see not only the differences but also the mixing. But how can we speak of mixture within the framework of the counter-notions of "difference" and "identity"? I myself do not believe that solid notions like "difference" and "identity" are suitable for talking about the *dynamic process* of interculturality. It is better to speak of "mixing" and to consider how this "mixing" takes place.

From this view point, I would like to speak today about the "*uniqueness*" of the world.

## 1. Neologisms and/or the Borrowing of Notions in Intercultural Encounters

Even in Europe, the modern notion of "*science*" is a fairly recent development. In Japan, it was introduced only at the end of the 19th century. Japan was long influenced mainly by China and Korea. Japan officially opened its doors to the West in 1868, and from that time, the main outside influence on Japan has come from the West. Near the end of the 19th century, Japanese thinker *Amane NISHI* (西周: 1829-97) translated the word "science" as "科学"[1], using Chinese characters (which Japan imported from China in the 5th century). Before Nishi's translation, these characters seem to have been used as a short expression for "科挙(之)学"[2], which means "learning in preparation for the Chinese civil service examination". The focus of these studies was to learn the classical texts, and the purpose of study was to get a job, rather than to search for "truth". "学" (學) originally referred to the place where boys went to learn: that is, a "school".

---

1 He translated the word "philosophy" as "哲学", with *Yukichi FUKUZAWA* (福沢諭吉:1835-1901).

2 There are some different writings for "科挙": "科擧" or "科举".

Nishi himself used the word "科" in the sense of "discipline" and "学" in the sense of "research". By his definition, "科学" was a collective name for the specialized disciplines that strived for knowledge of the truth[1].

The concepts of "objectivity" and "object" were also introduced to Japan about this time. We know that these words have a complicated history, even in the West. This history relates to the so-called "invention" of "subjectivity" and the "subject". *Michel Foucault* (1926-84) describes the formation of the subject under the panoptic system and in relation to the act of confession. *Jonathan Crary* shows its role in the development of the "sciences" and also its relationship to changes in social interest[2]. I will go back to Crary later. In any case, we should remember that the word "subject" originally referred to something "lying under", and that the word "object" referred to something "laid over" it.

Now, in East Asian culture, there was no concept of "subjectivity" and "subject" or "objectivity" and "object", at least in the epistemological sense. Therefore a pair of new words or neologisms were coined: "主観" (subject) and "客観" (object). Originally, "主" means "host" and "客" means "guest". ("観" means "seeing".) But it was and is difficult to express the whole scope of Western "subjectivity" and "objectivity" with these Chinese characters, so "主" and "客" are combined with other characters to express other meanings. For example, "主語" is used for the subject in the grammatical sense. "主体" is used for the subject in the practical sense. "主題" is used

---

1 In the Japanese tradition, "学" as learning is not only the learning of classical texts but also of technology. In the era before 1868, the idea of "和魂漢才" was widespread. It means "Japanese soul plus Chinese technology". Upon learning that Western technology was stronger than Chinese technology, the motto was changed to "和魂洋才", or "Japanese soul plus Western technology". Thus the purpose of science for the Japanese was never "pure knowing", but technological innovation for practical purposes. This is also related to the historical and world-political situation of Japan at this time. Japan had to make itself strong in order to avoid colonization by the West, such as that witnessed in the Opium Wars of the 19th century. This necessity led to strenuous efforts to become an "advanced" country. One needs to understand conditions like these in order to understand how science is accepted and developed in specific situations. But even this view of the Japanese understanding of science presents a problem: Is it possible to keep one's old soul while adopting a new and foreign technology? I believe that it is impossible.

2 Jonathan Crary, *Techniques of the Observer*, MIT Press, 1992.

for the subject as "theme", and so on. As for the meaning of "subjection" (in the sense of "lying under"), it is impossible to express this with the character "主". Normally, the idea of "subjection" is expressed with the character "従", which is in fact an antonym of "主". "主従", for example, means "master and servant".

There are similar complications with "object". Although "object" in the practical sense can be expressed as "客体", "objective" in the sense of "purpose" requires another word: "目的". For "objection" – in the sense of "opposing" or "disapproving" something – we normally use the expression "異議." "Object," "objective" and "objection" have common roots in most European languages, but they are expressed differently in Chinese characters. There are always gaps of understanding between cultures, because different cultures and different languages have different networks of meaning that come into play, even when they are trying to talk about the same thing.

Concerning "truth", there is an important notion in the East Asian tradition. We use the character "眞" (真) for "true" or "truth". There are various interpretations regarding the formation of this Chinese character, but one interpretation[1] says that this character is formed by putting "匕", which refers to the dead and which is the original form of "化" (which means "change" or "mutation"), together with the upside-down form of "首", which means "neck" or "head". According to this interpretation, the character "真" means that "there is no more change because of death". Here, "truth" lies outside change and outside of time. It is "atemporal". There are other interpretations as well[2]. Even within the same culture, different interpreta-

---

1 *Shizuka Shirakawa* (白川静: 1910-2006) criticizes this interpretation, which appears in *The Origin of Chinese Characters* (説文解字), which was completed in A.D. 100. 1500 years had already passed after the formation of Chinese characters, says Shirakawa. The materials cited by the author 許慎 were only 500 years old at most, after the characters had undergone many changes. Shirakawa himself referred to much older material that was discovered in the 20th century. According to Shirakawa, the interpretation of 許慎 was influenced by the thinking of the Later Han era (25-220).

2 Another interpretation says that this character is formed by combining "匕" and "鼎", and that the former is a "spoon" (as in the modern character for "spoon": "匙"), and the latter a vessel with three legs. The whole character indicates a

tions arise when history is long and tradition is old. We can also see this in Heidegger's interpretation of truth in the West. In any case, there was and is a notion of truth in East Asia, although it is not identical with that of the West. If we were to encounter a culture with no idea of truth at all, could we understand it or could it understand us? In any case, the fact that there was a notion of truth in East Asia, however different from the European notion, played an important role in the acceptance and development of Western science.

Concerning the European notion of "culture", we are told that it derives from "colere", an agricultural notion that refers to the tilling of soil. The notion of culture is normally positive, even when used by Hannah Arendt, who was very critical of everything. But we should not forget that the word "colonialism" also derives from "colere".

In China and Japan, culture is translated as "文化". But what do these characters mean? There are several interpretations, but the most interesting one says that "文" refers to the "tattooing of the living body" or " 文身" ("身"means "living body"). In ancient times, newborn babies were ritually tattooed, as well as young men who came of age. A tattoo was an appeal to the gods to activate the "life" of a person. "Life" is represented by the characters "生" and "命". Of the two, "命" means not only "life", but also "destiny" or "mission". "Life" in this sense is something that is given by the gods as a destiny, and the ritual of tattooing was intended to activate this life. A tattoo was something striking or beautiful that would capture the attention of the gods so that they would visit the person. Tattooing was, so to speak, a "phenomenalizing" or "making present" of the living body.

The living body functioned as a medium between humans and the gods, and between humans and other humans. Tattooing reinforced this function. It also "identified" the tattooed person as belonging to his culture. The tattooed person no longer belongs merely to nature. The tattooed body is the mutation of the natural body into a cultural body. I believe that all of our ways of seeing, of living, of thinking, and so on, are "tattooed" by our culture in some sense. We are all "culturally tattooed beings" or "incarnations" of culture.

---

vessel being filled with a liquid, using a spoon. In this case, "truth" is "fulfillment".

This interpretation alerts us to the important relationship between the living body and culture itself. But even those of us who use the word "文化" often "forget" this relationship. Nevertheless we can hear and see the relationship in the word and in the Chinese script. An etymological explanation can also help us "recall" what we have forgotten. This kind of "forgetting-recalling" occurs not only *intra*-culturally, but also *inter*-culturally.

East Asian people know that their present cultures have been strongly influenced by Western culture. Western culture has also been influenced by East Asian culture to some extent. For example, the importing of Chinese porcelain led to the development of the famous porcelain of Meissen. Importing is important. Without Japanese "Ukiyo-e", Jugendstil art would have been different. Although we should be wary of "Orientalism" (and also of "Occidentalism"), we can say at least that cultures are not "pure". They are always influencing and communicating with each other. We should always recall this. There are many other matters that we need to recall. Mutual understanding is difficult, because there is so much to recall and it is easy to forget. When we learn something, we forget something. Nevertheless, difficulty is not impossibility.

Does what I say include anything new and interesting for you? I hope so. Comparing things, learning new facts, recalling old facts – this can be interesting. But this kind of talk is still two-dimensional, if not trivial. It lacks an important consideration: the idea of viewpoint. My talk so far has been made from an "objective" viewpoint, or from a "third person perspective". We must go on to consider, philosophically and phenomenologically, the problem of viewpoint.

## 2. The Viewpoint of Phenomenology

The fact that there are many differences between cultures motivates us to "compare" them, just as I have done. I think comparison is necessary. But what does it mean to "compare" scientifically? Does it mean to compare things as they "are", "objectively", and to deal with them without bias? We should also ask: *Who* compares? This question evokes the problem of the "subject": that is, the one who sees in order to compare. Here, we encounter a basic premise of phenomenology: *it is impossible for anyone to see something from outside his or her original circle of vision*. That is, it is impossible to see "objectively" in the strict sense of the word. Everyone is already "culturally tattooed", even in that original circle of vision. A purely "natural" person might be able to observe all cultures fairly and objectively. But there is no such thing as a purely natural person, and if there were, he or she would not be able to recognize cultures as such, in order to compare them[1]. *A culturally tattooed viewpoint is inherent in thinking about culture.* This is an indispensable condition for the experiencing of culture, but it also makes a completely disinterested comparison of cultures impossible[2]. This is the case for comparison within a culture, and it is even more so for intercultural comparison. I would like to develop this insight, but for that purpose, it is necessary to clarify the idea of the "viewpoint" in phenomenology.

The "phenomenological reduction" is an important and well-known part of the phenomenological method. Some people think the reduction is a reduction of everything to consciousness. Is this true? If it is true, what exactly does it mean: to reduce something to consciousness? More inquiry is needed.

Husserl used the term "transcendental subjectivity". This sounds metaphysical, but Husserl says it is not a metaphysical construction but "a sphere of experience-based research" (Hua VII p.349[3]).The notion of "subjectivity" is a product of Western thinking. Jonathan Crary demonstrates this point well in his research. He begins with the idea of the "camera obscura" (cf. fig. 1), then goes on to discuss so-called "scientific" studies of subjectivity (although Crary refers to the "observer" instead of using the term "subjectivity") (cf. fig. 2). Subjectivity is interpreted as being more or less independent of the world, especially with regard to the phenomenon of the "illusion", which does not correspond to any "objective" thing. But a dualism of subjectivity and objectivity is always implied. The subject is inside the camera obscura and the objects are outside. In this scheme, *the subject is a prisoner of his subjectivity*. This analogy of the camera obscura is very naïve, but even very recent discussions of the problem of "qualia," whose "objective" correlates are so hard to find, relate directly to

---

1 We should recall that Hans-Georg Gadamer made similar observations about "prejudice".

2 What if we were to pluralize the "observer-subject" who compares? It might be better than just one observer. But how many observers would be enough to ensure disinterestedness and objectivity?

3 Hua: Edmund Husserl, *Husserliana*, Martinus Nijhoff & Kluwer Academic Publishers.

this dualism of subject and object (cf. fig. 3). This is precisely the point that Husserl criticized.

In a prelude to phenomenology, *Ernst Mach*, who also used the word "phenomenology", used an interesting illustration in a book of his[1] that Husserl also read[2]. It shows how we see the world from an original circle of vision (cf. fig. 4). The important point here is that *the circle is not closed. We are not prisoners* in it, whereas the analogy of the camera obscura makes us prisoners. Husserl's most fundamental insight was that it is impossible to "see" this circle from outside the circle, although we "believe" that an outside does exist. This way of thinking that it is possible to step outside, or "transcend", the circle was criticized by him as a "transcending act of thinking" (Hua II p.39) or as a "transcending interpretation" (Hua X p.5). Husserl says that we always stay inside the circle, although we believe that the outside exists "objectively". How is this possible? This was the problem Husserl wanted to solve. In order to do so, he proposed that we suspend our belief in the outside and go back to the original circle of vision. This is the "epoché" and the "transcendental reduction". In this context, Husserl also suspends the way we see the original circle "objectively". Our way of seeing the original circle is "subjective" in the sense that it is "not-objective". Nevertheless, subjectivity has the capacity to constitute *a belief in "objective" Being* that "transcends" the circle, and this is what Husserl calls "transcendental subjectivity".

Inside the circle, everything appears in a perspective manner. Take the example of a trapezoid or parallelogram. According to Husserl, there is an a priori structure of representation, whereby things are represented "by-means-of" or "through" certain appearances. For example, we see a square "by-means-of" or "through" a parallelogram. The parallelogram is an "appearance" of the square. We cannot see the square without the "appearance" of the parallelogram. We can see the thing itself, but only "by-means-of" or "through" its appearance. The square itself and its appearance as a parallelogram are in a relationship of correlation. This struc-

---

1 Ernst Mach, *Zur Analyse der Empfindungen*, Jena 1886.

2 This does not mean that the origin of the term "phenomenology" as used by Husserl came directly from Mach, nor the original idea of the "original circle" of vision. I believe that at that time in Vienna, there was a common tendency of thought that led to Husserlian phenomenology as one of the results. But I use Mach's drawing to illustrate a major aspect of the phenomenological method.

ture is found within the original circle of vision, without transcending it. Husserl named this the *"universal a priori of correlation"* (Hua VI p.169f. fn.).

Which do we "see"? The appearance or the thing itself? In a sense, we can say that we see the thing itself, and not the appearance. For example, this "pen". But how about this "duck" (cf. fig. 5) – or is it a "rabbit"? We always see something "*as* something". We "interpret" it in the widest sense. The "*as* something" can be different for each person, and the individual way of seeing is sometimes merely idiosyncratic, but more often, it depends on his culture. This could easily lead to a personal or cultural relativism. But what is the former "something"? Is it "objective", while the way of seeing it is "subjective"? Although we talk about the former "something" as something very solid, it is possible to talk about it only "regressively", after seeing it "*as* something". We grasp the thing and its appearance together, in correlation[1]. According to Husserl, all our experiences – namely perception, imagination, language, etc. – have the same structure of correlation.

The "*as* something" (or "appearance") of perception corresponds to "meaning" in language. For example, the meanings "evening star" and "morning star" relate to what is normally called "Venus" in the way that "perceptual sense"[2] relates to "what appears". Therefore we grasp "Venus" by-means-of linguistic meanings and "what appears" by-means-of perceptual sense.

Because there is such a universal and therefore exchangeable structure between language and perception, we can "communicate" with each other about perception "by-means-of" the meanings of an *intra*-cultural language. One person may say that something "appears" as a "trapezoid" to him or her, and the other may say that it "appears" as a "parallelogram". But we can understand that the two expressions both point to the same "square". "Trapezoid" and "parallelogram" are compatible as "two appearances of the same thing" in this case. In many cases, such differences of

---

1 Husserl found in later years that the former "something" has a "genetic" structure. According to this analysis, it has *in itself* the tendency to appear as the latter. But it is precisely in this genetic process that the cultural moment functions.

2 The integration of perceptual senses is called the "noema".

"appearance" will contribute to a richer understanding of "what appears" instead of detracting from it[1].

How about intercultural communication, where there is no "common" language? If all experiences[2] have the same structure, and if all of us have at least *the experience of perception*, we can "generalize" this structure at the level of intercultural communication. The differences of appearance will usually be greater than in intra-cultural communication. Nevertheless, if we understand the other's voice to be *speaking a language*, and therefore as something that has "meaning", this will provide a starting-point for mutual understanding. (If we don't understand the voice as language, communication is hopeless.) And indeed almost all the worlds' cultures are already communicating with each other.

Husserl originally developed his insight of a "universal a priori of correlation" as a way of explaining the relation between different kinds of experiences, such as perception, imagination, language, and so on. But his insight also shows us the possibility of intercultural communication, although it is more difficult. The reason for the added difficulty is that no meaning is isolated. Each meaning is entangled in a network of many meanings, which Husserl referred to as a "horizon". In order to know the meaning of a word or character, we need to know its horizon, as I have tried to illustrate with my examples of Chinese script. But difficulty is not impossibility. The "fusion of horizons" is possible, and it is always occurring.

## 3. The Problem of the World in Phenomenology

In order to think more about the world from a phenomenological point of view, let us go back to the starting point. We normally think of the relationship between subject and object along the model of the camera obscura. We think that every subject has before him or her not only the appearances of things, but also a world. This would mean that there are (plural) worlds, because there are plural subjects. Is it so? But we have already

1 Of course, meanings can also be incompatible. Some combinations of meanings belong to the realm of "impossibility". This means that there is a framework of "possibility", which Husserl also investigated.

2 In Husserlian terminology, we should speak of "acts" instead of "experiences". An "experience" is a kind of "act". An "act" is that in which something appears.

confirmed (phenomenologically) that this way of thinking is very problematic. After all, we see everything inside our original circle of vision. And we also know that the plurality of appearances does not contradict the singularity of the thing that appears. Should we say then that the plurality of the appearances of the world does not contradict the singularity of the world itself? Does this mean that the single common world is the biggest "thing" or biggest "object" in our circle of vision? This is the second important problem.

What is an "object", when we say that it has "objectivity"? This is such a difficult notion that there is no word in my language that corresponds exactly to the term. In any case, an "object" should be independent of the subject. It should "be" in itself. The Being of things in themselves is a condition for objectivity. In contrast to this, the "meaning" or "sense" of an object depends on subjectivity. But here a question arises. How can we – the subjects – who cannot transcend the original circle, have a notion of objectivity that assumes the possibility of seeing something independent of a viewpoint? Objectivity so conceived has at least two layers: it is a Being that is acknowledged subjectively, and it is also acknowledged intersubjectively or interculturally.

Objects of perception (which have "real Being") have one moment of objectivity, and this way of Being is expressed in European languages in the "indicative mood". In contrast to this, objects of imagination or fantasy have "quasi-Being", which is generally expressed in the "subjunctive mood". This means that the latter have no objectivity[1]. Phenomenologically, however, even the possibility of "real Being" must be explained within the original circle. Husserl's answer to this problem is not very clear. Nevertheless we can find suggestions in his analyses of real Being and quasi-Being. I will quote one example: "Something fantasized is always something temporal; for example, each sensuous phantasm is the fantasy of a sensuous object, and intentional temporality is a part of this merely intentional object. The fantasized object is regarded as temporal and time-

1 This is actually incomplete: we accept also, for example, the Being of transcendent numbers such as "π" of which the Being is not "real" but "ideal". This Being does not accept variations of tense. It rejects "it was" and accepts only "it is", whereas real Being accepts "it was". Nevertheless, both real and ideal Being are expressed in most European languages in the indicative mood.

determined, as continuing in time, although its time is quasi-time." (EU p.196[1]) For example, Snow White belongs to quasi-time. So do the Little Mermaid and Sinbad. But the time of each of these fantasies has no relation to the others. And each quasi-time has no unity with other quasi-times. But for us, there is a special time that is integrated as "one". For something to have real Being, this something must be related to *this one time* and be located in it. Quasi-Being, on the other hand, is located in quasi-time and has no relation to *the one time*. Only things located in *the one time* can have real Being. This one time, which enables real Being, is a condition of possibility of objectivity and is called "objective time". It is unique, whereas there can be plural quasi-times.

Once more, if something belongs to this "unique" time, it is acknowledged as having "real Being". If not, it is said to have mere "quasi-Being"[2].

Husserl develops this idea further to the idea of the "uniqueness of the world". Husserl says that the world is "temporal". This does not mean that the world is *in* time, but that the world and time are "one". Therefore, an object located in the world is acknowledged to have "real Being". If it is not, its "real Being" is denied and it is called an "illusion", or it is said to have mere "quasi-Being".

How about the "Being" of the world itself? It is impossible to locate the world in the world. If someone says that there "is" another world, we should ask: "Where is it then?" The answer must be "somewhere". But the word "somewhere" is meaningful only when the possibility of a location, namely "the world", is already given. (This is also the case with "sometime".) In this sense the idiomatic English expression "where in the world?" contains a truth, since everything must be somewhere in the world. Another aspect of this is, that, while it is possible for plural things to exist in the world, it is not possible for plural worlds to exist within that world. The world must be "one" and "unique" (Hua VI p.146)[3]. Consequently, the Being of the world is totally different from the Being of things. It is pre-given

1 EU: Edmund Husserl, *Erfahrung und Urteil*, Felix Meiner 1985.

2 The ideal object is ubiquitous in both objective and quasi-time. This ubiquity is a kind of Being — an ideal Being. But ideal Being does not transcend all time. It appears *in* time. In this sense, it is also a kind of temporality: an omni-temporality, not an a-temporality, to be precise.

3 The "uniqueness" of the world was for Husserl an important issue of his original idea of "metaphysics".

without a location for itself. Husserl says that there is a difference "in principle" between "the manner of the consciousness of the world" and "the manner of the consciousness of things". (cf. Hua VI p.146) *The unique Being of the world is a condition of possibility for the real Being of all things.*

The unique world is there, as a condition of possibility, but it remains unthematized by us. Only by being un-thematic can the world play its role. When it is thematized, as "this world" or "that world", it is localized as a kind of "thing". When this happens, the world as unique world must be enlarged in order to locate the thematized world within its boundaries. The enlarged unique world itself is again un-thematic. This means that a thematized world is not a "true" world, but a kind of object within the true (enlarged) world. I said earlier that the Being of things is a condition for objectivity, and now I can add that the unique Being of the world is the condition for the Being of things.

4. The Problem of the World in Intercultural Phenomenology

According to Husserl, the notion of "objectivity" relates not only to the world but also to "intersubjectivity". That is, to be "objective", something must be accepted by "every" subject. Within the notion of intersubjectivity, we can differentiate between *intra*-cultural and *inter*-cultural subjectivity. Although the distinction is only an "ideal" one, we can use it to analyze the concept of "mixing". Thus, we can continue the discussion of the previous section and ask: How does the unique world relate to the problem of the two kinds of intersubjectivity?

In a shared cultural world, we see the "homely" Other who is familiar to me as a "comrade". We acknowledge that he or she has a personal "world". But both the Other and this personal "world" are located within our common (intracultural) world. Certainly this "world" of the Other has aspects unknown to me. But this is also the case for other ordinary things. Even the most ordinary things – a pen, for example – has aspects unknown to me. Of course there is a basic difference between the unknown aspects of a pen and the unknown aspects of the Other: while the aspects of a pen can be known to me, those of the Other cannot, in principle. But even if we know that the Other has, in principle, an unknown side, this does not threaten the unity of our (intracultural) world. The Other's "world" is implicitly located in our common world, together with everything else. We do not normally thematize it, but even when we do, it is smoothly integrated into our world. The world remains comprehensive and comprehensible.

But what happens in the case of an intercultural encounter? Husserl says that the world has plural "stages". This idea of "stages" is important for the analysis of intercultural encounters.

What happens when we encounter not a homely Other, but a foreign and strange one? Husserl says that at the moment of the encounter, such an Other is entirely beyond our comprehension (Hua XV S.432). In this instant, we know that this Other is beyond our understanding and we also realize, at the same time, that our own understanding was limited. This strange Other does not belong to our comprehension, is not a comrade. He or she is simply "foreign". The limit of the comprehensiveness of our own world is known *thematically* to us at this time. Phenomenologically speaking, the difference between "home" and "foreign" (or "nearness" and "farness", "familiar" and "alien") becomes decisive.

The foreign Other is "uncanny", at least for the subject who has been culturally tattooed in a specific but different way[1]. We can run away from the foreign Other. But we can also try to understand him or her. We often find that the ways of seeing, of living, of thinking, are different from ours. The difference is unlike the differences we find in our own intracultural world. This strange Other "appears" as someone who comes from *outside* our world, as someone who has a world – a "foreign" world – of his own. But the appearance of this Other and this foreign world is seen from the viewpoint of our own world. This is when we notice that our world is in fact "our" world. This is when we first thematize it as a "home world". The home world is thematized because of the appearance of a foreign world. Homeliness is thematized because of foreignness. They are thematized as counterparts and, in this sense, as a "pair"[2]. Then "comparison", which derives from the Latin *par* (or "pair"), occurs almost inevitably. But in order to be "compared" properly, both must be dealt with on the basis of a shared world. Indeed, both "worlds" are now located in an (enlarged) world, although this enlarged world is not yet thematized. But the important point

1 But something uncanny can also be attractive. In any case, for the culturally tattooed subject, the uncanniness of the Other is factually inevitable.

2 This means that a total thematization is impossible. Only the concerned parts are thematized (as counterparts).

here is that the two "worlds" which are now being compared are no longer unique worlds with no location.

In attempting to understand the foreign Other, we learn to see the "foreign" from the viewpoint of "home". But the latter is a condition of possibility (and also a source of difficulty) for understanding the former. Despite the difficulty, we can attempt to understand the foreign. Once we understand the foreign, we gain the ability to see things and ourselves "through" (or "by-means-of") the Other's way of seeing. This is an important ability for interculturality. But the starting-point for that understanding is always our (culturally tattooed) homeliness, which means there is an "asymmetry" between our way of seeing the "foreign" and our way of seeing the "homely".

When we attempt to understand both the foreign and homely, the world enlarges itself implicitly in order to include both. But when a new "foreign" appears, the previously enlarged world is thematized again, as a home-world of a different level. But there is still an asymmetry between home and the foreign, because the original cultural tattooing of the home-world carries on, unthematically, into the enlarged world. Here again, we cannot transcend our original circle of vision, but we usually forget about this impossibility and think that we are looking at home and the foreign "objectively" so to speak.

I would like to reformulate the problem here using the concept of stages. There are at least three "stages" to the world. At first, the world is simply "unique". I call this the "primal-singular" stage, when the world is completely un-thematized and "incomparable". But then we experience the difference between our "home world" and a "foreign world", and both worlds are thematized and become "comparable". This is the second stage. But these two worlds are found to be located in one larger world. This world might be called the "supra-singular" world, which is once again un-thematized and "incomparable". This is the third stage. The movement from stage to stage is a continuous whole, but not smooth, because the subject is culturally tattooed. There is always some asymmetry. Every time we encounter something unknown, something uncanny, a "world-quake", so to speak, occurs. And encounters with the foreign are not one-time occurrences. They happen successively. Our unique world continually experiences such world-quakes and continually rebuilds itself. This is also the case with the notion of objectivity. A static or stubborn objectivity is impossible. Objectivity also experiences the same kind of movement. This is not a negation of objectivity. It means that we need a more dynamic and modest notion of objectivity.

## Conclusion

I would like to recapitulate the main points of my presentation. At the beginning of this presentation, I posed the methodological question of intercultural comparison. It led us to question the viewpoint of the subject/observer who makes the comparison. In this context, I presented the insights of phenomenology regarding the impossibility of comparison from outside the viewpoint. We see everything from inside the original circle of vision, where something appears. This led us to the relation between "appearance" and "what appears", which is mainly a matter of "things" and how they appear to us. This led to the problem of the world, where these things are. The world is and must be unique, but this uniqueness is problematic when we consider the situation of intercultural encounter. A "mixture" or fusing of worlds occurs, but we see that this mixing is already at work in intraculturality. Let me add now that, from the very beginning, it is never possible to divide cultures clearly. They are part of the movement of a "unique" world that is continually moving between three stages. Even intercultural comparison is part of this movement.

But this movement of the world is always experienced within the original circle. *Who* experiences it? *Who* compares cultures? We might give a *pro-visionary* answer and say that it is the *I*. But we must then ask what this I is, how it relates to the world, and how it relates to the Other. It is not a "merely subjective" I. It is not at all the I in the normal sense, even if it is named the I[1]. What role does it play in interculturality? Our asking does not end yet at all.

---

1 How different is this I from the normal I? In any case, it "extends" itself with the enlarging movement of the world, since even such a world is experienced by the I. In this special sense, it has an "extension", unlike the Cartesian I. It partly overlaps with the Kantian I of apperception, because this I relates to the unity of the (enlarged) world. But it has a "genetic" formation. It does not constitute the world in a one-sided manner. Rather, in a sense, it is due to the world that it occurs. Its relation to Others, who appear both as comrades and as strangers, is more complicated. This indicates a special double movement. But one of the most important functions of the I is somewhat parallel to that of

I hope that my presentation has contributed somewhat to clarifying the methodological problems of scientific research into interculturality. But the asking is more important than the answer. Asking can move something, while the answer stops it, and only something that moves can resonate with the world-movement. I hope that my asking has moved something in you.

---

the "house" or "home", which, because of its "door", can be open or closed to the Other. In this context, some related Chinese characters are illustrative ("家", "客", and "主", "住"). A "家" (house) was a holy place, which relates to the holy animal sacrifice "豕" (which in this case meant a dog, although the form was similar to and is often confused with a pig). And "羊", which means "sheep", was also such a holy sacrifice. The Chinese characters which correspond respectively to "good" and "justice", "善" and "義", both have "羊" as a component. This is also the case with "美", which corresponds to "beauty". These all relate to the idea of "death" (as sacrifice). As mentioned in the main text, the Chinese character for "truth", or "眞", also relates to "death". What does this suggest? Our life in general is inseparable from death, since the ideas of "truth", "good" and "beauty" are central to the way our lives relate to the world and to Others. What is the role of the I then? We should consider at least the two Chinese characters, "我" and "吾" for "I", which I believe contain some hidden suggestions toward a new idea of the I.

Kambiz Badie and Maryam Tayefeh Mahmoudi

# Capturing Insight & Wisdom through Making Resonance between the Patterns of Differing Knowledge Systems

## 1. Motivation behind the Present Topic

Biological system (plant of body) is subject to transformation at both physical and chemical levels and such transformations are expected to lead subsequently to both organic (structural) and functional changes in the body. Since the performance of the organs with regard to a variety of biological scenarios is a matter of importance, it would be crucial to investigate the possible scenarios to treatment for inhibiting the possible damages. The following scenarios may exist in this regard:

(i) Based upon a treatment, the damaged structure would be improved.
(ii) Based upon a treatment, the damaged structure would be controlled (not to be damaged any more).
(iii) The performance of an organ can be controlled in an overall way, despite any possible growth in the ongoing damage.

Coming to the philosophy of medication, it is obvious that the very medical systems being used to manipulate problematic situations in the body, try somewhat their best to pay attention to the above scenarios in some manner. Naturally, based upon the basic philosophy behind each system, the status of this attention would be different. The systems discussed above can be regarded as kinds of knowledge systems including their peculiar reasoning and action patterns for treating disease/disorder situations.

Since no meta-theory can exist explaining the symbolic inter-relations between two different medication systems ( as two differing knowledge systems), contexts of experiencing these systems in terms of applying them to real scenarios of diseases/disorders, may be regarded as appropriate media through which the related reasoning as well as the action patterns, can be checked to yield finally an appropriate framework for mapping from the main reasoning propositions in one system onto a range of allowable action propositions in the other one.

Our main point here is that, provided that a diagnosis ( and the corresponding treatment) can be regarded more and more reliable, if it is simultaneously approved by different knowledge systems, and in the meantime the expert of a knowledge system ($KS_1$) ( who is familiar with the reasoning and action patterns in $KS_1$) believes that the treatment pattern in another knowledge system ($KS_2$) can be equally reliable, it would then be reasonable to make use of the experienced scenarios as a means for configuring the action patterns ( in $KS_2$), which can at the same time be justifiable for the expert of $KS_1$. This necessitates a process for monitoring such scenarios together with the related reasoning patterns in $KS_1$ and at the same tome the corresponding action patterns in $KS_2$. Having accomplished such a process, a new situation is faced, according to which the expert of $KS_1$ would have the confidence to confront with certain action patterns in $KS_2$ that can equally function reliably in response to his/her reasoning pattern.

Such a process provides us a chance to assess the reasoning pattern suggested by a knowledge system somewhat by the action pattern in the other knowledge system, to increase its level of confidence in some way. In case of any discrepancy it might be important for the specialist in $KS_1$, to change his/her reasoning pattern and the corresponding action pattern in $KS_2$, and repeat this process until the stage where the level of confidence to be looked for becomes sufficiently satisfactory. At this stage, both the specialists of $KS_1$ and $KS_2$ get aware of the fact that an action pattern may exist in one of the knowledge systems that can equally be acceptable for both of them. (Refer to Table1). In the meantime, one can claim that the two knowledge systems have been functioning cooperatively to assure emergence of a secure action pattern (Figure1(a) and (b)).

The afore-mentioned process can be particularly effective in the situations where the action propositions in one knowledge system can be particularly favorable ( with regard to a variety of attributes) compared to another knowledge system. If we consider the case of medication, where treatments are expected to be as favorable and low- risk as possible respecting a variety of attributes, the significance of such a process gets obvious.

Table1. From the reasoning pattern in a knowledge system onto the action pattern in another knowledge system

| Phase No. | Function of the Phase |
|---|---|
| Phase1 | Suggesting the reasoning pattern for a certain problematic situation using the propositions in $KS_1$ |
| Phase2 | Finding the equivalence for the reasoning pattern using the propositions in $KS_2$ |
| Phase3 | Checking the equivalence using the reasoning pattern in $KS_2$ |
| Phase4 | Going back to Phase1, if the suggested reasoning pattern is not satisfying enough, otherwise terminating the procedure |

## 2. What Methodology Can Support the Desired Process?

Taking into account the above discussion, it becomes clear that a proper association between the reasoning pattern in one knowledge system and the action pattern in another knowledge system offers an opportunity to the medication specialist to select the efficient solutions with less side-effect. Such an association can be viewed as a kind of indirect interaction between the two systems, which is only realizable by means of a connectionist framework [1,2]. It should be noticed that, in contrast with symbolic frameworks that are equipped with logic of reasoning, connectionist frameworks have the capability to make correlation between chunks of experienced information with no emphasis on logic of reasoning. Both bidirectional associative memory (BAM) [3, 4] and adaptive resonance theory (ART) [5,6,7,8], as two well-known connectionist frameworks, are workable in this regard (see figure 1(a)).

Bidirectional associative memory may be helpful in the sense that, through triggering the concept of reasoning pattern belonging to $KS_1$, the concept of an action pattern belonging to $KS_2$ would be established. Here, both patterns can be represented in terms of appropriate propositions to be observed in the structure of the connectionist framework in terms of appropriate nodes. Contexts should also be represented in terms of sets of appropriate propositions, which are to be equally observed in the framework's structure.

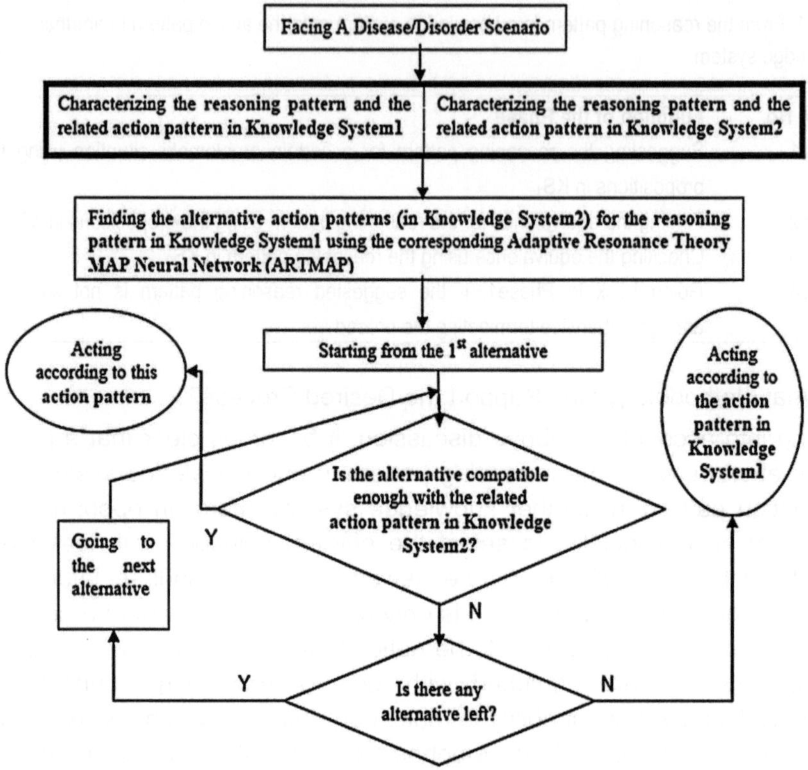


Figure 1(a): Assessing the reasoning pattern in a knowledge system by the action pattern in another knowledge system

Obviously, some criteria are required to assess the status of an action pattern's emergence based on the status of energy level at the corresponding nodes. With regard to Adaptive Resonance Theory (ART), reasoning patterns in $KS_1$, represented in terms of appropriate propositions as the input features, are clustered based on the idea that appropriate weights ought to be established for the links connecting these features to the prototypes at the output of ART network.

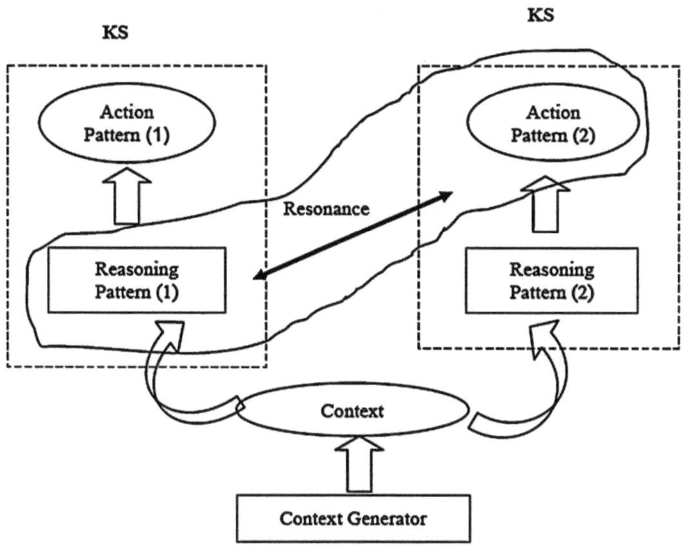


Figure 1(b): Co-operative functioning of the two knowledge systems to assure the emergence of a proper association

In this way the status of similarity between a new reasoning pattern (as the feature vector) is decided not only by the internal product of this feature vector and the corresponding weights of the connections, but also by the vigilance factor which has been pre-determined for each prototype to assure the quality of the affiliation of the related vector to the candidate prototype. Taking this point into account, once a new pattern (as a feature vector) is assigned properly to the corresponding prototype, resonance would occur in the sense that the weights of the corresponding connections in the network are strengthened, while those belonging to the non-relevant connections are weakened. Such a process is believed to be helpful because a high number of reasoning patterns, which may differ from each other partially, can be grouped into only a limited number of clusters that can later be used meaningfully for the subsequent process of decision-making. Association in this way can make sense between the input reasoning patterns belonging to $KS_1$, and the prototypes of the output action patterns belonging to $KS_2$. Such an association can gradually become more and more significant, if a large number of previously-experienced scenarios of observing associations between the reasoning patterns ( in $KS_1$) and action patterns ( in $KS_2$) are taken into consideration. In our approach, we make use of ART network to show the way the reasoning patterns in one knowledge system ($KS_1$) can lead to emergence of possible action patterns in another knowledge system ($KS_2$).

## 3. Basic Concepts in Adaptive Resonance Theory (ART)

### 3.1 Motivations for Memorizing the Previously-experienced Pattern in terms of Appropriate Clusters

An important point with regard to the experienced patterns is the very similarities which stand for their closeness toward certain characteristics. Such closeness can be an excuse to believe that certain clusters (or groups) of experienced patterns would better be finely associated with similar (classes of) representative prototypes. In this way, memorizing the experienced patterns would make sense through memorizing (preferably a limited number of) representative prototypes. The representative prototypes memorized in such a way have the capability to contribute to the subsequent decision processes (such as classification process) that are primarily considered for the experienced patterns. Coming back to the role of reasoning patterns, one can see the situation where the experienced reasoning patterns in $KS_1$ are memorized in terms of a limited number of prototypes, so that when a new reasoning pattern (the reasoning pattern for a new problematic situation) is considered, based upon the prototype triggered, a subsequent process would be activated to yield the wanted action pattern in $KS_2$. Obviously, the higher quality of memorization, the higher quality of final association would be. This necessitates a kind of on-line process for updating memories according to which the memorized prototypes can be updated based on new arrivals of the input patterns, until the stage where they can get stabilized at appropriate modes. i.e. a process which can be realized in a type of network functioning on the ground of adaptive resonance.

Figure2 illustrates a schematic for ART network. As it is seen from this schematic it consists of two layers; a comparison layer and a recognition layer composed of neurons, a vigilance parameter, and a reset module (from Wikipedia, the free encyclopedia). The vigilance parameter has considerable influence on the system: higher vigilance produces highly detailed memories (many, fine-grained categories), while lower vigilance results in more general memories (fewer, more general categories). The comparison layer takes an input vector (a one-dimensional array of values) and transfers it to its best match in the recognition layer. Its best match is the single neuron whose set of weights (weight vector) most closely matches the input vector. Each recognition layer neuron outputs a negative signal (proportional to that neuron's quality of match to the input vector) to each of the other recognition layer neurons and inhibits their output accordingly. In this way the recognition layer exhibits lateral inhibition, allowing each neuron in it to represent a category to which input vectors are classified. After the input vector is classified, the reset module compares the strength of the recognition match to the vigilance parameter. If the vigilance threshold is met, training commences, otherwise, if the match level doesn't meet the vigilance parameter, the firing recognition neuron is inhibited until a new input vector is applied; training commences only upon completion of a search procedure. In the search procedure recognition neurons are disabled only one by one by the reset function until the vigilance parameter is satisfied by a recognition match. If no committed recognition neuron's match meets the vigilance threshold, then an uncommitted neuron is committed and adjusted towards matching the input vector.

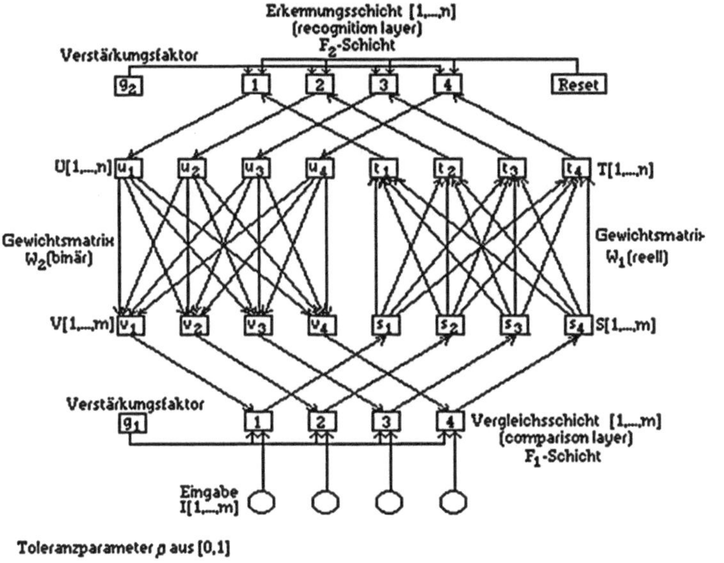


Figure 2: ART Network

4. Our Proposed Approach to Employing ART Network

We start our discussion with two pre-suppositions as follows:

*Pre-supposition 1*: Each reasoning pattern in $KS_1$ consists of a number of propositions, which are represented in terms of individual inputs, to which a variety of possible values within a certain interval can be assumed based on the status of these pre-positions.

*Pre-supposition 2*: Each action pattern in $KS_2$ consists of a variety of propositions, to which individual ART networks are assigned.
The outputs of these networks stand for the possible status of the related propositions in the corresponding action pattern in $KS_2$.

Taking the above pre-suppositions into account, the main phases in our approach can be summarized as follows:

*Phase1*: The objective of this phase is to group the feature vectors consisting of the propositions belonging to the reasoning patterns, in the form of appropriate prototypes as the outputs of a simple ART network.
Regarding this, a simple ART network is used.

*Phase2*: The objective of this phase is to re-organize the prototypes obtained in phase1 through checking their validity by means of the information on the right status of the corresponding propositions belonging to the related action patterns in $KS_2$. Regarding this, an ARTMAP network is used [5,7,8].

Since for each individual proposition belonging to an action pattern in $KS_2$ an individual network is used, the final result of making association (between a reasoning pattern in $KS_1$ and the corresponding action pattern in $KS_2$) would be a combination of the outputs of these networks, Figure 3(a) and (b) illustrate such a process.

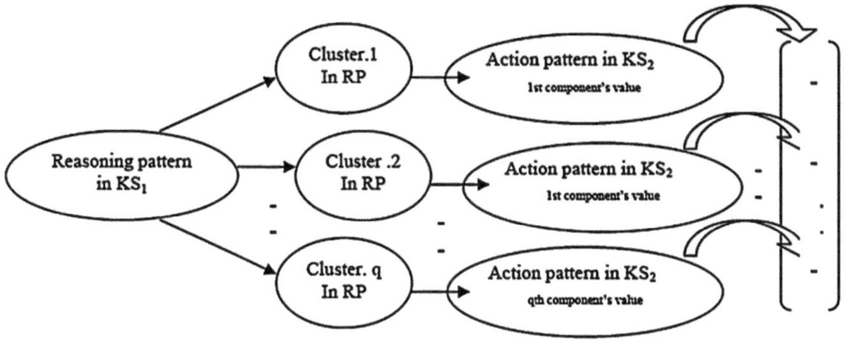


Figure 3(a). From reasoning pattern in $KS_1$ onto the structure of action pattern in $KS_2$

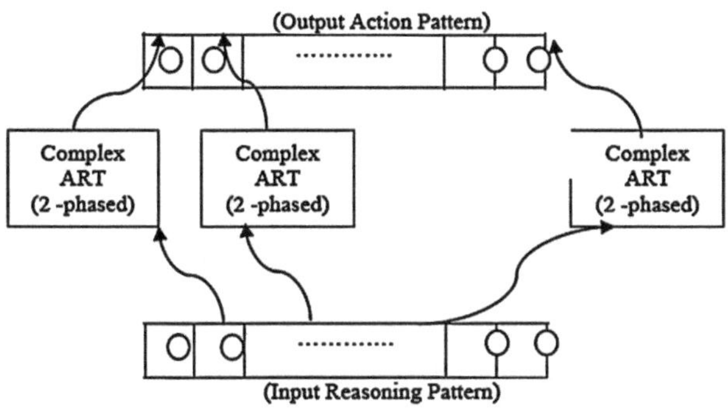


Figure 3(b): Combination of the outputs of networks as the result for association

Coming to the nature of medication problem, various layers exist each including its own propositions. These layers can be conceptualized as follows:

1. Layer of Disease/Disorder's Context: It stands for the symptoms/signals of a disease/disorder.
2. Layer of Structural/Functional Change: It stands for the possible structural or functional changes which, may occur in anatomically significant parts at different levels. Let say, for instance, the structural/functional

change in the organs such as brain, kidney, lung, heart or liver that can be conceivable for certain symptoms/signals observed from the patient.

3. Layer of Reasoning Pattern: It stands for the rational reaction of expert's mind toward a certain context appearing in terms of appropriate propositions. Let say, the pattern of reasoning to be suggested by a doctor, when he/she observes symptoms/signals from the patient, or certain structural/functional change in certain organs of this patient.
4. Layer of Action Pattern: It stands for the pattern of treatment that an expert may exhibit once he/she arrives into a certain pattern of reasoning.

It is interesting to notice that, from a cognitive view-point a kind of association exists between each two consecutive layers. Let say, an expert's mind may be associated with some qualities of structural/functional change, once a certain disease/disorder with certain peculiarities is faced, while such qualities of structural/functional changes may in turn make his/her mind be associated with a certain reasoning patterns that itself can be a motivator for the expert to converge into a certain action pattern with certain characteristics. As is seen, a variety of different associations can be established between these layers, as illustrated in Figure4.

Two points should be considered in this respect as follows: 1) Although the layers discussed here seem to be in common for most of the medication specialists; let say most of the experts try in some way to have first an estimation of a "structural/functional change" in anatomically significant parts, and then establish their "reasoning pattern" for these changes based on their knowledge and finally converge into an appropriate "action pattern" to cover their reasoning pattern, based on the cultural background of the expert and his/her individual mental experience (that can be expected to be almost unique), some additional metaphors can emerge for them, each showing up in terms of an individual layer. In this way, one can expect for a higher number of associations to be learned by the expert.

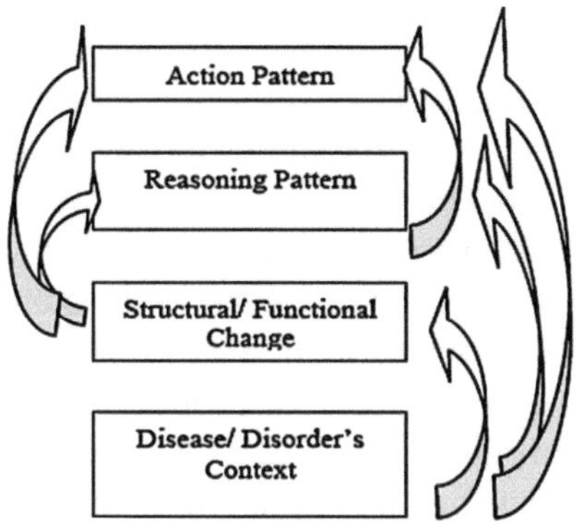


Figure 4: The entire associations to be learned between the layers in medication problem

To upgrade the performance of an association, in addition to the medication expert's reasoning pattern, additional information regarding the disease/disorder's context (based upon which the expert has arrived into the reasoning pattern) as well as the structural/functional change can also be used.

The later can be provided via a direct association with the disease/disorder's context either by making use of an artificial ART network, or asking the expert's opinion about the structural/functional change. Figure5 illustrates a configuration where the final action pattern in $KS_2$ is produced under collaboration of the other 3 layers.

The main reason for the increase in association performance in this configuration may be due to a kind of fusion effect [9,10] that tries to compensate for the probable deficiency in a direct association of the reasoning pattern with the action pattern, through considering some complementary (though redundant) information components in the input of the ART network. These components themselves have been a ground for constituting the reasoning pattern as the prime input. Let say, despite the fact that information on both the disease/disorder's context and structural/functional change are redundant with respect to the reasoning pattern as the prime input, their redundant presence in the input of the ART network, strengthens the effect of the expected association which leads to the desired action pattern.

## 5. Claim of Capturing Insight & Wisdom through Association

### 5.1 Claims for Insight

Having established association between the combination of disease/disorder's context, structural/functional change and the reasoning pattern (belonging to $KS_1$) on the one side and the action pattern (belonging to $KS_2$ ) on the other side, the question here is whether or not it could be possible to attain an insight respecting the relations between the two knowledge systems ($KS_1$ and $KS_2$). In a classical symbolic way of thinking, the association between two sets of propositions can be made on the ground of a number of rules, where each rule describes how certain combinations in one set can be associated with certain combinations in another set. Having these rules calls for presence of a meta-theory to be used as a ground for making implications between the rules' conditions on the one side and their actions on the other side. Since such a meta-theory does not exist (mainly due to the fact that the two knowledge systems come from different orientations of thinking), the only approach left to making associations is the connectionist framework that was already discussed. This connectionist framework has the capability to make some hypothetical knowledge with symbolic nature, regarding the relation between its input and its outputs. Let say, the way this framework reacts toward certain structures in the input in terms of certain propositions in the output, may stand for certain rules that indicate the inter-relations between the two knowledge systems in some way. When the variation in these rules gets high, we will face a situation according to which an insight can be claimed to have been established between the two knowledge systems. The rules extracted in such a way can subsequently constitute a suitable reference for the researchers in the field of comparative medicine to take their pace for measuring the symbolic relations between the two systems.

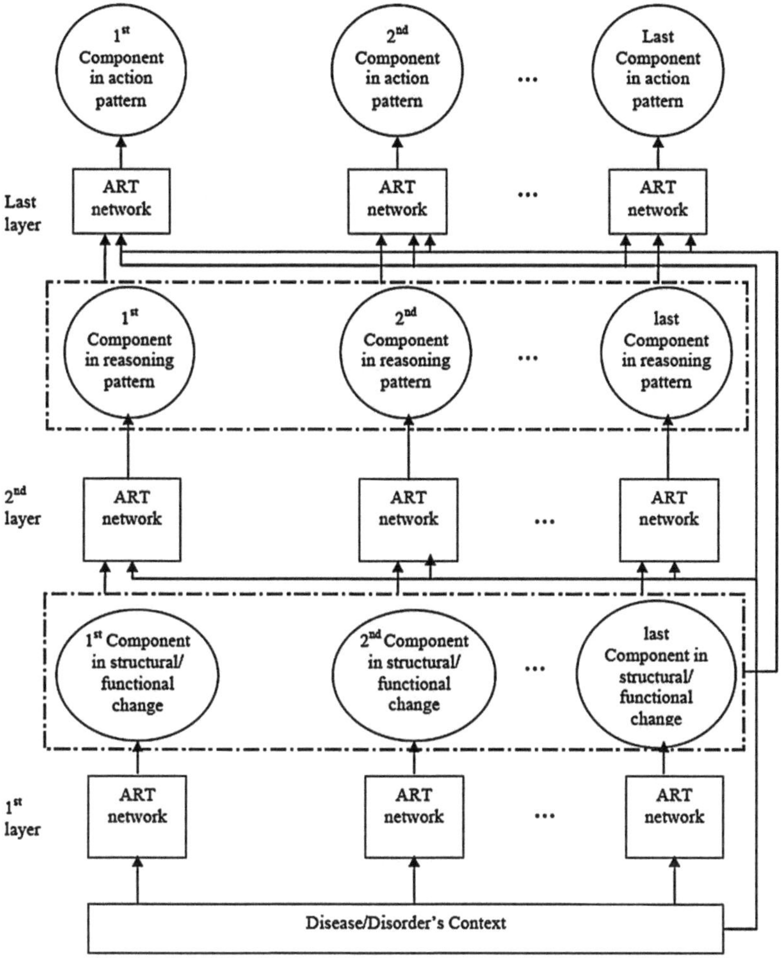


Figure 5: Upgrading the performance of association via considering redundant information components in the input of the last layer of ART networks

## 5.2 Claim of Wisdom

The term wisdom is mostly used in the case where a reasonable and in the meantime effective utilization of knowledge with regard to an ongoing situation is considered [11, 12, 13]. Let say, the value of wisdom goes back to the fact that how valuable using a certain chunk of knowledge can be assessed for a certain situation. Wisdom is in this way meaningful since it assures the way chunks of knowledge can be employed for handling a certain problematic situation. Wisdom is in many cases empirical, in the sense that no meta-theory can prove its validity, and it is mostly a wide spectrum of past experiences that can take the responsibility of this validation.

Coming back to the issue of making association between the reasoning pattern in a knowledge system, and the action pattern in another knowledge system, which is based on a kind of resonance between the related patterns, wisdom can be meaningful where selecting a particularly effective & low-risk choice for treatment (from the viewpoint of a variety of parameters) is a matter of question.

Let say, provided that a certain action pattern in a knowledge system, like a pattern of treatment, can equally yield the same effect as the one belonging to another knowledge system, but its cost and side- effect is reasonably lower than the one of the later, it would be an indication of wisdom to make use of the former as the alternative for treatment. The relation between resonance and wisdom can thus lie in the fact that the association established on the ground of resonance, makes a suitable medium for comparing the action patterns in the two systems, which in turn would tell us how the corresponding knowledge can be utilized in an efficient matter. This is exactly the goal being pursued by wisdom. Figure 6 illustrates a schematic where the association between the set of reasoning propositions and a context on the one side, and the action propositions in another knowledge system on the other side, can be finally viewed as a kind of wisdom for the corresponding specialist.

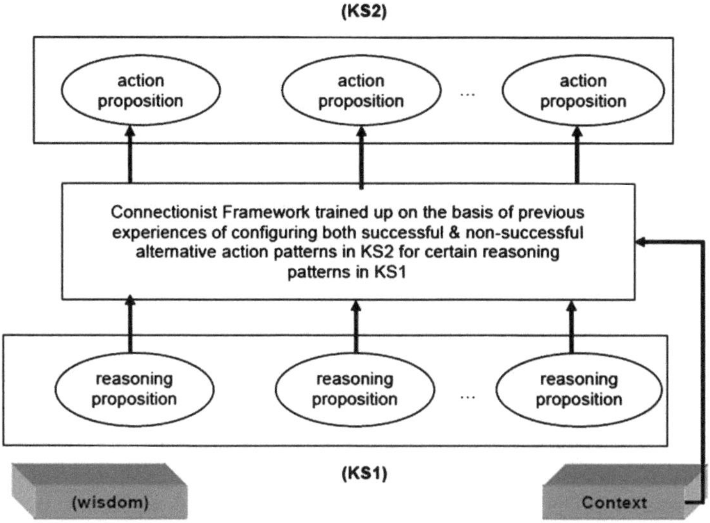


Figure 6: A simple schematic of viewing wisdom for a specialist

## 6. Concluding Remarks

It was discussed in the paper that, establishing associations based on making appropriate resonance between the patterns in two differing knowledge systems, like two differing medication systems, has the capability to yield finally a forum wherein the experts of both of the knowledge systems can capture insight into the inter-relations between the two systems on the one side, and wisdom on the alternative treatments with least side- effect on the other side. In our approach, we made use of adaptive resonance theory to establish the essential association in an appropriate manner, taking into account different layers for which intermediate associations based on local resonance can be meaningful. It was discussed in the paper that, establishing association in a multi-layer manner would lead to upgrading its performance mainly due to a kind of fusion effect that tries to compensate for the probable deficiency in a direct association of the reasoning pattern with the action pattern through considering some complementary (though redundant) information components in the input of the

ART network. Taking into account the afore-mentioned points, it becomes obvious that the proposed approach to making resonance between the patterns of two differing medication systems can be successfully used as suitable alternative for making adequate comparisons between the two systems by the time a pathological situation is faced.

References


1. D.E. Rumellhart, J.L.Mcclelland, "Parallel distribution processing: exploration in the micro structure of cognition", Cambridge, MA: MIT Press1.
2. D. E. Rumellhart, G. E. Hinton, and R. J.Williams, "Learning internal representations by error propagation," Parallel Distribution Process: Explanations Microstructure of Cognition, Vol. 1, pp. 318–362, 1986.
3. B. Kosko., "Adaptive bidirectional associative memories". Applied Optics Journal, Vol. 26, No.23, pp. 4947-4959, 1987.
4. B.Kosko, "Bidirectional associative memories", IEEE Transactions on Systems, Man and Cybernetics, Vol.18, No.1, pp.49-60, January/February 1988.
5. G.A.Carpenter, "Distributed learning, recognition, and prediction by ART and ARTMAP", neural networks, Neural Networks, Vol.10, pp.1473-1494, 1997.
6. G.A. Carpenter, S.Grossberg, D.B.Rosen, "Fuzzy ART: Fast stable learning and categorization of analog patterns by an adaptive resonance system", Neural Networks, Vol4, pp.759-771, 1991.
7. G.A. Carpenter, S. Grossberg, N. Markuzon, J.H.Reynolds, D.B. Rosen, " Fuzzy ARTMAP: A neural network architecture for incremental supervised learning of analog multidimensional maps", IEEE Transactions on Neural Networks, Vol. 3, pp.698-713, 1992.
8. G.A. Carpenter, "Distributed Prediction and Hierarchical Knowledge Discovery by ARTMAP Neural Networks", Knowledge-Based Intelligent Information and Engineering Systems, Springer Berlin / Heidelberg , Vol. 2773, 2003.
9. D.R.Radev, "A Common Theory of Information Fusion from Multiple Text Sources- Step One: Cross-Document Structure", http://www.sigdial.org/workshops/workshop1 /proceedings/radev.pdf.
10. B. C. Gruber-Geymayer, A. Klaus, K. Karner, "Data Fusion for Classification and Object Extraction", In: Stilla U, Rottensteiner F, Hinz S (Eds) CMRT05. IAPRS, Vol. XXXVI, Part 3/W24 , Vienna, Austria, August 29-30, 2005.
11. A. Zuckerman, "Wisdom", Hachette Australia Pub., 2008.
12. R.J. Sternberg, "Wisdom: Its Nature, Origins, and Development", Cambridge University Press, April 27, 1990.
13. D.J. Soccio, "Archetypes of Wisdom: An Introduction to Philosophy". United States of America: Wadsworth Publishing, 2006.

Jeremy Rosenbaum Simon

# Intercultural Medicine and Western Philosophy: Constructing a Home for the One within the Other

## 1.

If you ask most people about the logical relationship between Western and traditional Chinese medicine (TCM), they will probably say that they cannot both be true. The two seem to be describing such different physical systems that they cannot both accurately represent the functioning of the human body. What will likely also follow, for a Westerner, is that since Western medicine is so well confirmed scientifically, or at least, its biological basis so well understood, it is Western medicine that accurately reflects the real world, with TCM being false.

This at least is what the realist, who believes that science's goal is to provide an accurate picture of the underlying structure of the natural world, will say. Either the human body has meridians or it does not, and thus Western medicine and TCM cannot both be true. (Of course they can both be false.) A constructivist about medicine, who believes that our medical categories – diagnoses, organ systems, etc. – are social constructs that have no basis in any underlying natural world, could grant equal validity to both TCM and Western medicine, but it is a validity that many would find inadequate. After all, it would seem to leave us with little reason to believe that either practice will reliably work.

These two options, realism and constructivism, dominate the dialectic in the analytic philosophy of medicine, and therefore, for an analytic philosopher, it would seem that at most one of the two medical systems we are discussing can be true in a realist sense. Recently [Simon 2008], however, I have begun developing an account of the metaphysics of (Western) medicine based on the constructive realism (CR) of Ronald Giere [Giere 1988, 1999].[1] I believe that, properly understood, this constructive realism

1 This is to be distinguished from Fritz Wallner's version of constructive realism.[Wallner 1997] Although it is not a coincidence that both philosophies are called "constructive realism, Wallner's approach to the relevant matters strike

yields an account of medicine that leaves room for both Western medicine and TCM to potentially be true in the realist sense of representing the underlying natural order of the world. Meridians may be as real as marrow, and chi as real as neural impulses. Thus, in addition to providing the best understanding of the nature of medicine and its relationship to the world, I believe that CR provides a fruitful and non-exclusionary basis for understanding the relationship between Western medicine and TCM.

In what follows, I want to show how this is. I will begin by describing Giere's CR. After this, I will show how it applies to Western medicine, describe how it can be applied to TCM, and finally draw some conclusions.

Before beginning, I must point out that whereas my understanding of Western medicine comes from many years of training and practice as an allopathic physician, my knowledge of TCM is only that of an interested layperson. I am therefore not in a position to undertake in this paper the same reconstruction of TCM as a constructive-realist practice as I have done for Western medicine. The best I can hope to do at this time is show how CR applies to medicine in general through the example of Western medicine and then indicate without giving a concrete example, how, despite the difference in methods and concepts, the same approach can be applied to TCM. I believe that this will be adequate to show the value of the current approach for philosophers interested in TCM.

2.

The purpose of developing a constructive-realist medicine was to help us understand the ontological nature of the entities medicine deals with, especially diseases. When we say that a patient has cystic fibrosis, say, to what sort of entity are we referring with "cystic fibrosis"? For reasons that we cannot get into here, I believe that both the realist and constructivist approaches are unsatisfactory in this regard. I therefore turned to CR to create a successful (I believe) alternative account of the nature of disease entities.

Before seeing what a constructive realist approach to medicine looks like, let us review the theory in the form in which it is most completely developed – Giere's exemplar, classical mechanics. To see how scientists

---

me as being closer to van Fraasen's constructive empiricism than to Giere's constructive realism.

understand the world, that is, what claims they make about the world, Giere says, the best place to look is in textbooks, where this understanding is passed on to a new generation of scientists at the beginning of their training. These texts, Giere notes, open with a presentation of Newton's laws. They do not, however, proceed to deduce anything from these laws, as we would expect if these laws really constituted the fundamental content of mechanics. Rather, after this initial presentation of Newton's laws, these textbooks generally proceed with chapters discussing different forms of the force function F = (ma =) f(x). For example, this section of the text might begin with a chapter on the simple linear harmonic oscillator, governed by the equation F = -kx, followed by examinations of the pendulum, where F = -(mg/l)x, and the two-body system, where $F = Gm_1m_2/r^2$.

What, Giere asks, is the relationship between the systems described by these textbook presentations and governed by these equations and the real world? Factors such as ignoring the angle of swing in the pendulum equation and the assumption of uniform gravitational fields assure that the equations do not precisely describe any actual real-world system. Rather than precise descriptions of (part of) the real world, Giere claims that systems described in mechanics texts, such as the harmonic oscillator, are *models*, "*abstract entities* having all and only the properties ascribed to them in the standard texts" [1988, 78, emphasis in the original]. Although Giere does not spell out what he means by "abstract entity," the context makes his meaning relatively clear. Abstract entities exist not in the physical world but only in the realm of thought. One example of abstract objects Giere gives is linguistic entities (although models are not linguistic entities) and other might be numbers and universals, at least under a Platonist interpretation. With this understanding of models, what we would then say about the linear harmonic oscillator is that it is simply an abstract system obeying F = -kx (with "F" interpreted as force and "x" as position). One consequence of this approach to the linear harmonic oscillator is that we should now think of it (and other textbook models) as a constructed entity, since it has been (abstractly) constructed by physicists to meet the specification F = -kx.

Having seen what models are, we can turn to their relationship to the outside world that physics purports to deal with. According to Giere, this relationship is one of *representation*. Scientists use models to represent the real world through models' role in theories. For Giere, theories describe the real world through two main components. In addition to models, scientific theories comprise "theoretical hypotheses." The role of these hypotheses is to assert relationships of representation between models and particular real-world systems. For example, classical mechanical theory would have an hypothesis stating that the model named "a pendulum" represents a particular component of grandfather clocks, and that the "two-body system" model represents the earth and the moon. But what does it mean to represent in this sense? For Giere, models represent real-world systems via similarity. Of course, since all objects are similar to each other in some way, there must be some parameters governing the similarity of model to real-world system if the former is to be considered to represent the latter. Therefore, beyond stating that a certain model is similar to a given real-world system, theoretical hypotheses add that they are similar in specified respects and to a specified degree. For example, the hypothesis governing the earth-moon system might be: "The positions and velocities of the earth and moon in the earth-moon system are within five percent of those of a two-particle Newtonian model with an inverse square central force."

This is the basic structure of Giere's system as applied to mechanics. Before moving on to medicine, there are two more features of Giere's models we should consider. First we have identified Giere's CR as a realist account of science, as Giere himself does. In what respect is it realist? The realism here is modal realism – CR accepts that the real world has a modal, or causal, structure. Therefore, for a model to be acceptable within CR, its modal structure must reflect the real world's modal structure. In other words, modal claims the model makes such as that the position of the harmonic oscillator at $t_1$ varies depending on its position at $t_0$, are taken to be true of the real-world system the model represents and are not considered mere artefacts of the process of making abstract models of the real world. CR is thus realist because it claims that not only does the world have an underlying causal structure, but a scientific theory is true only if it in fact reflects that underlying structure.

The second point to address, which is especially important for what will follow in our application of CR to TCM, is the question of choice of models, or theories. Scientists can construct endless models. How do they choose which to use? Most such constructions fail to meaningfully represent anything and can be immediately discarded, assuming they are created in the first place. However, it may remain the case that several models appear to potentially represent a given real-world system, such as the human body. Scientists must then decide which model to use in their theory. As a primary criterion, they will likely assess how well the models fit reality. Scientists are likely to prefer a model that consistently gives results within one percent of the observed real-world values to one that gives results within five percent. However, there is a second criterion. Scientists need to be able to use models to understand the behavior of real-world systems. Therefore, depending on the tools available to them and the cognitive strategies they prefer, scientists may find a less accurate model a more useful tool in this regard that one that is more accurate. It may be that the more accurate model's mathematics is too complex, or it represents things arithmetically to a society more used to geometric thought. Whatever the issues, when confronted with multiple models for the same system, scientists will choose the one that best suits their needs overall, considering both accuracy and preferred cognitive strategies. Of course, often the choice will be implicit, with the geometrically minded community not even developing the arithmetic model. However, the important implication here is that there is no unique set of correct models and real entitles associated with them. There may be two conflicting systems of models that represent the behavior of the human body, both of which are equally true. An analogy may be helpful here. The underlying structure of the world may be compared to a large board cut like a jigsaw puzzle and reassembled. There are a limited number of ways, but no one unique way, to divide this board into smaller blocks of pieces. Scientists are, as it were, looking at the board and trying to predict what shape pieces they can break the board into. If the piece they try to break off comes off cleanly, they have succeeded in making a model, as it were. Two different groups of scientists may, successfully, break the board down into very different shaped pieces.

It is important to note that this discussion only describes one aspect of Giere's overall account of science, and that only partially. I have done justice neither to its complexities nor its problems and have omitted many features of Giere's account. Such discussions, however, will not be necessary for our current purposes.

3.

Let us now see how to apply this concept of model to (Western) medicine. Our exemplar, rather than the harmonic oscillator, will be cystic fibrosis (CF). To provide some background, especially for those who are not familiar with this clinical entity, I want to provide a brief summary of a standard textbook treatment of CF, in this case, abstracted from *Harrison's Principles of Internal Medicine* [Boucher 2006].

The chapter starts with an explanation of the molecular basis of the disease. Patients with CF have a disorder of one of the ion-transport pumps in their cell membranes (the CFTR protein). As a result of one or two of hundreds of mutations in "cystic fibrosis gene," the CFTR protein is either not functioning properly or absent altogether. After presenting this background, the chapter goes on to explain how this defect manifests itself clinically. As a result of disordered ion-transport, chloride and sodium build up within cells, and this metabolic disarray leads to various physiological ill effects, many of which can be attributed to the thickening of mucus and other secretions as a result of the imbalance of ion flow. Most dramatically, CF patients have poor pulmonary function and are particularly prone to pneumonia. The other two most commonly affected organ systems are the gastrointestinal tract, where patients may suffer from obstructions, malabsorbtion of nutrients, and pancreatitis, and the reproductive system, with sterility in many men and delayed puberty in both sexes. Next, the chapter discusses the diagnosis and general prognosis of CF. Finally, we learn that there is at present no treatment for the underlying disorder in CF, although individual problems like infections and intestinal obstructions can of course be treated directly, and attempts to develop gene therapy to provide properly functioning CFTR proteins to patients are underway.

Let us now try to understand cystic fibrosis as a Gierean model. Cystic fibrosis would then be an abstract entity with all and only those features attributed to it above. However, we must determine which part of this description of CF we consider the description of its model. I do not believe that the entire chapter constitutes a description of the model. Medicine is different from physics in this regard. Unlike physics textbooks, which merely need to teach students how to think about the world abstractly (no basic physics text will include instructions on how to build a satellite), medicine texts also need to teach their readers how to apply their knowledge to the real world. Thus, in addition to models, they will explicitly include what we would call linking hypotheses and perhaps other real-world information as well. What we need, to identify a model for CF, are the parts of the chapter that describe a system that can develop over time, and describe it in such a way that we can both understand and to some degree predict the system's behavior. Furthermore, since we are developing an abstract model, this information should be abstracted away from any real-world system and not simply consist of empirical statements and observations. Under these guidelines, we arrive at the following interpretation of the cystic fibrosis chapter. The description of the ion-transport system provides the essential model of CF, describing both the state and the development of the (abstract) system in question. However, the description of the ion-transport system does not stand alone. In classical mechanics, the explicit description of the model encompasses all features of the model. In medicine, however, models include an implicit addition. The explicitly described model of the part of the body most affected by a given disease needs to be understood as embedded in an otherwise unspecified human being, or, more precisely, in an abstract system representing the physiology of a generic human being. In our case, this amounts to pointing out that a cell by itself cannot have cystic fibrosis. It is only when we take into account the effects of the cell's altered ion transport mechanism on various organ systems that we have CF. Thus, an adequate model of CF, one that actually represents the clinical entity in question, must incorporate models of these systems, at least implicitly.

I do not want to discuss here the role of the chapter's genetic account of CF in our constructive realist reading. It is complicated and not relevant to our concerns here. Suffice it to say that I do not consider it part of the CF model. Moving beyond biophysics and biochemistry, then, we need to provide a constructive realist reading of the descriptions of the organic and systemic pathology, natural history, and treatment of the disease. The model cannot comprise these, since particular patients who we want to say have cystic fibrosis can differ from what is described in these sections too greatly to be encompassed by the phrase "within specified respects and specified degrees." Therefore, the simplest way to read these sections is not as part of the model, but rather as presenting empirical observations a clinician will want to know regarding the development of the real-world systems (patients) that are represented by our medical model. This mixing of theoretical model and empirical observation in a single discussion reflects the dual purpose of medical textbook. They not only give physicians a general understanding of disease and medicine, but also need to provide practical information for dealing with actual patients.

Finally, we must discuss the section on diagnosis. This too, is not part of the model. However, it does have an important role in a constructive realist reading of the chapter. Particular acts of diagnosis are essentially the formulation of a theoretical hypothesis: "This patient, to high degree, is similar in the relevant respect of having a particular ion-transport system, to the model disease cystic fibrosis." A discussion of diagnostic methods and criteria in a medical text is therefore a guide to forming the theoretical hypotheses without which a constructive realist science is incomplete.

4.

The general CR account of (Western) medicine, then, is as follows. Ontologically, a disease is an abstract entity, a model that specifies the structure of part of an otherwise unspecified human organism. When we combine this disease model with our model of general human physiology, we can make predictions about how a real-world system represented by this joint model, that is, a person with the disease in question, should develop over time and in response to various environmental impacts. To the extent that a given disease model, by embedding the relevant causal structures, allows us to accurately predict and affect the clinical course actual patients, that model will represent a (constructively) real disease.

I think it is clear how this approach to medicine can be applied to TCM as well, and be applied to TCM side by side with Western medicine. In CR, particular diseases, as well as physiological systems like the respiratory system and the nervous system, are real, and make the assertions of (Western) medicine true, because they embed a description of the causal structure of the world accurately enough for doctors and others to make successful predictions about how real-world systems will develop under different circumstances. These models do not, however, successfully embed these causal structures by describing them in a uniquely correct way. Rather, the models provide scientists and doctors with an intellectually congenial way of making accurate predictions. This accuracy is evidence that the models embed the requisite causal structures and are therefore real. The possibility of there being more than one model, or system of models, that embeds the requisite causal structures for a given physical domain is explicitly acknowledged.

It is therefore possible for two groups of investigators, especially two groups from different cultural and intellectual backgrounds, to confront the same scientific domain, in this case the functioning, and especially, malfunctioning, of the human body, and develop entirely different, even incommensurate, models to accommodate and comprehend that domain. In the case of Western medicine, as we saw, the account consists of disease models combined with, or embedded in, a model of human physiology built around systems such as the nervous system, the respiratory system, etc. These components, however, are simply features of the given model, not necessary parts of any correct account of the world. They are part of the abstract representation of the human body constructed by Western physiologists, not part of the uniquely correct representation of nature of the world.

The scientists who constructed the system of TCM confronted the same domain of experience and constructed an entirely different model, or set of models, to organize it. I say domain of experience and not body of experience because it is possible that, in addition to non-Western cognitive patterns, one of the features that may have lead TCM to a different model of human physiology and illness may have been experience with physical events and capabilities Western medicine was not directly exposed to, e.g., the abilities of certain martial arts masters. At any rate, as I said above, I am not familiar enough with TCM to tell a story about it as I did above with Western medicine. However, with some trepidation I will attempt to give a very general outline of such a picture.

Although in the discussion of Western medicine above we considered disease models primarily and models of general physiology only incidentally, I will start here by describing (again, only generally) the TCM model of human physiology. One would begin by opening a textbook of TCM, such as, for an English speaker, Kaptchuk 1983 or Maciocia 2004, 2005, 2008, and seeing how it describes the functioning of the human body. What one would find, I gather, is a description of the twelve Zang Fu organs, jing, chi, and shen, meridians, and a few other components. The structure and behavior of these systems (for lack of a better word) would be described, and furthermore, we would learn how they relate to each other and interact to result in an independently functioning organism.

Since we are constructive realists, however, we must not take these descriptions to apply to any physical entities. Rather, just like Giere's harmonic oscillators or our CF above, they are accounts of abstract entities, models, existing only in the minds of those scientists (and practitioners) who have studied and understood them. We need further linking hypotheses (which may or may not be explicitly stated in the texts) to tell us how to relate these models to real-world entities. Thus, for example, one linking hypothesis may tell us that jing is, or, more precisely, the model named "jing" in the text represents, (a component of the) fluids that one observes, e.g., when an incision is made in the body, as well as in other circumstances, such as after ejaculation. Another will state that chi is the energy one observes the body producing under particular circumstance. (I am sure that neither of these is quite right, but I trust that it is a close enough approximation to illustrate the point.) Finally, there will be a linking hypothesis that the higher level model composed of the interacting models for the Zang Fu organs, jing, shen, etc., represents a human organism.

The final component of a constructive realist account of TCM is an assertion that it works. That is, once we understand, via linking hypotheses, how the models of TCM relate to human beings, we can use our understanding of the models and their behavior to predict and understand the behavior of human bodies, since, TCM asserts, these models represent, to within a certain adequate degree of accuracy, the behavior of actual human bodies under various circumstances.

If TCM understood pathophysiology like Western medicine, I would now have to describe a TCM model of disease, along the lines of the model of CF described above. However, to the extent that I understand it, TCM does not seem to make use of notions of diseases and diagnostic entities in the way that Western medicine does. Rather, when a patient has a complaint, the TCM practitioner carefully examines the patient, looking for signs of imbalance in the patient. Thus, they will examine the pulse, the tongue, the hair, etc., and deduce from there, as well as the patient's responses to various questions in the history taking, where in the patient there is an imbalance, and what the nature of the imbalance is. Various therapies can then be prescribed to correct the imbalance and make the patient healthier.

Given this description of TCM diagnostics, it seems that there will be no models of disease of the sort we described for Western medicine.

However, this does not mean that we cannot understand TCM practice through the perspective of CR. For a constructive realist, the TCM practitioner understands how the models TCM uses to represent the body will react to various hypothetical external insults. Furthermore, he knows how these changes will manifest themselves in the parts of the model which correspond to the externally accessible diagnostic aspects of the human body (pulse, tongue, etc.). Using this knowledge, and the fact (presupposed by the practice of TCM) that these models accurately represent real human bodies, i.e., work, the practitioner can work backwards from the external signs and known environmental insults to internal imbalances in the patient, and then, finally, know which therapies will affect the patient in the desired way.

Before moving on, I want to make two points. First, although I have just described TCM as lacking diagnostic entities, nothing in what follows hinges on this. If one understood TCM as recognizing diagnostic entities one would complete the CR picture of TCM taking the relevant texts, perhaps Maciocia 2008, and abstracting the disease models from there, just as we abstracted a model of CF from Boucher 2006. However, both because it seems to me to be a more accurate representation of the practice of TCM, and because I do not have enough understanding of TCM to undertake even a sketch of a TCM disease-model, should it even be advisable, I have presented a CR account of TCM without diagnoses.

Second, it may be objected by those who know the TCM literature better than I do that much of what I evidently suppose is to be found in TCM texts is not there at all, and that much of the knowledge of, say, interpreting physical findings is passed on through direct instruction and not in texts. Even if this is true, this lack of text would not affect our CR account of TCM either. Written texts make it easier for the outside researcher to reconstruct the models, but oral instruction can be treated as a virtual text. Of course, understanding the models may not be simply a matter of transcribing the teacher's words onto paper, as much of the information may be transmitted by exhibiting real patients (just as it is in Western medicine). However, an underlying model will still be there. The case would be analogous to a physics student who was taught physics not through textbook models but by being shown (in one lesson) various (low friction) pendulums and told, look how these pendulums all swing with a fixed period proportional to their length. This would transmit the same knowledge, based on the same underlying model, as the textbook chapter explaining that the force function of a pendulum is $F = -(mg/l)x$.

5.

Now, why would one want to take a CR approach to TCM? One answer is that it gives the most accurate account of TCM's claims about the world, just as it does for physics, medicine, and indeed all sciences, by which I mean practices that seek to allow us to understand and potentially influence the functioning of the physical world. Of course, this is a mere assertion on my part, as I have not, and will not, here do the work necessary to demonstrate this.

There is, however, another benefit to adopting a CR approach to TCM, one that I mentioned above and want to say more about here. If one is a constructive realist, one has no problem, in principle, saying that both TCM and Western medicine are true, or more specifically, that the entities they describe in their accounts of physiology and medicine are real. For, to a constructive realist, there is no unique true description of the world and set of real entities. To be real is to accurately reflect part of the underlying causal structure of the world. Any model or set of models that successfully represents a part of the world by accurately describing the behavior of that part of the world is a true description of the world and the entities represented by those models are real. There is no claim, or reason to believe, that there is only one set of models that can mirror a given domain, such as the functioning of the human body. Thus, different sets of people, especially if they are focused on somewhat different processes or features of the world, can create different sets of models to represent a domain. However, since if they both accurately represent the world they are both reflecting the same underlying causal nature of the world, the entities represented by the models of both systems are equally, and simultaneously, real.

Thus, if Western medicine is successful, the nervous system, lungs, and cystic fibrosis are real. If TCM is successful, meridians, chi, and the xin bao luo are real. If both are successful, then all of these are real.

It is important to note that although the entities of both Western medicine and TCM may be real, this does not mean that they can necessarily be integrated into a single system. Indeed, it is highly unlikely that this can be done. For, although all of these entities represent the underlying causal structure of the world, they do so using different cognitive strategies for approaching the world and organizing experiences. Thus, while both systems may cut nature at joints, these are unlikely to be the same joints, and thus the pieces from the different systems are unlikely to fit together with each other. To recall our jigsaw analogy, if TCM and Western medicine each had a copy of the board, the pieces Western medicine breaks the board into and the pieces TCM breaks it into would not fit together in most cases.

An important consequence of this probable incommensurability is that although, assuming both practices work, both TCM and Western medicine may be able to return a given patient to health, it could be counterproductive to use them in concert. For, though both practices will start with the patient at the same point (a given ill state) and aim to move him to the same point (health), they will usually take different routes to get there, following different causal pathways dictated by their different representation of the causal structure of the world. Thus, the two therapies, at any given time, may attempt to pull the patient in different directions, as it were, and thus interfere with each other. Even if there is no destructive interference, there is no clear reason to suppose that the two sets of therapies will move the patient to her destination quicker than either one by itself.

6.

Where does all this leave us? Nothing said above should be taken as an argument that TCM gives a true picture of the world. Everything that I have said thus far about TCM could be said, mutatis mutandis, about any other healing practice, such as homeopathy or witchcraft. In order for TCM or any other healing practice (including, of course, Western medicine) to be describing reality, its models must succeed in representing that reality. That is, it must work in treating patients.

There is, therefore, both a challenge and an opportunity here for TCM. The challenge is to provide evidence of its success. (Perhaps this challenge has been met. I am sure it depends on what type of evidence you insist on, something I will not even touch on here.) I should point out that this success does not need to be defined on Western medicine's terms, but can, to a large degree, be measured in the terms of the goals TCM sets itself. The object of TCM qua science is to represent the world in such a way that it can be understood and manipulated. Thus, if TCM's models allow TCM practitioners to manipulate the world in the way they want, i.e., achieve the goals it sets for itself, then these models have done all that we could ask of them.

The opportunity that arises from meeting this challenge is the potential for attributing reality to the entities of TCM – chi, meridians, etc. – in exactly the same way, and at the same time, as it is attributed to the entities of Western medicine or other sciences. TCM will not have to make (or rather, be perceived by Western philosophers and scientists as having to make) any apologies, accommodations or translations to Western systems. It will have established its own truth, thus constructing a home for itself in the West along side Western medicine.

References

Boucher, Richard. C. 2005. Cystic Fibrosis. In *Harrison's Principles of Internal Medicine*, 16th ed., Dennis. L. Kasper, et al., eds. New York: McGraw-Hill, pp. 1543-6.

Giere, Ronald. N. 1988. *Explaining science: A Cognitive Approach*. Chicago: The University of Chicago Press.

Giere, Ronald. N. 1999. *Science Without Laws*. Chicago: The University of Chicago Press.

Kaptchuk, Ted J. 1976. *The Web That has No Weaver*. Boston: Charles Tuttle.

Maciocia, Giovani. 2004. *Diagnosis in Chinese Medicine: A Comprehensive Guide*. Edinburgh: Churchill Livingstone.

Maciocia, Giovani. 2005. *Foundations of Chinese Medicine: A Comprehensive Text for Acupuncturists and Herbalists*, 2nd ed. Edinburgh: Elsevier Churchill Livingstone.

Maciocia, Giovani. 2008. *The Practice of Chinese Medicine: A Comprehensive Text for Acupuncturists and Herbalists*, 2nd ed. Edinburgh: Elsevier Churchill Livingstone.

Simon, Jeremy. 2008. Constructive Realism and Medicine: An Approach to Medical Ontology. *Perspectives in Biology and Medicine*. 51:353-366.

Wallner, Fritz G. 1997. *How to Deal with Science If You Care for Other Cultures: Constructive Realism in the Intercultural World*. Vienna: Braumüller.

Yishan Duan

# Medical Contents and Cultural Connotations of "Preventive Treatment" in Chinese Medicine

*Translated by Fengli Lan*

Abstract: Medical contents of "Preventive Treatment" can be summarized as "Three Preventions", i.e. "Preventing Illness from Occurring", "Preventing Illness from Progressing", and "Preventing Illness from Recurring". "Preventive Treatment" is an intensive reflection of the inherent awareness of hardship of the Chinese nation, and its cultural connotations mainly stress "thinking of danger in times of safety" and "nipping an evil in the bud".

What is the bounden duty of the medical practitioners? What is the tenet of the medical organizations? Confucius's evaluation on *The Book of Songs* (Shi Jing, 诗经) can be used to answer the above questions: "In one statement, take the preventive treatment".

Why? With the changes in the disease spectrum, the medical mode in the 21st century has transformed from the biological to the biological – psychological – social – environmental, and the emphasis has transformed from the mid-late stage of diseases to the entire period, especially to the early stage or before the occurrence of diseases. In other words, the center of the concern has been moved forward, from treatment to prevention, from diseased condition to the condition before the occurrence of diseases, and from disease to health, which indicates that "preventive treatment" has been forwarded as an important task to solve problems of human life and health since the ancient times. In the past two years, the idea of preventive treatment has been so popular in mainland China that many hospitals have set up special departments for providing such a kind of treatment. For example, centers of "Preventive Treatment" have been established in Shuguang Hospital and Yueyang Hospital of Integrated Traditional and Western Medicine affiliated to Shanghai University of Traditional Chinese Medicine.

1. Medical Contents of "Preventive Treatment"

The idea of "Preventive Treatment" in Chinese medicine originates in *Plain Questions* (Su Wen, 素问) and *Miraculous Pivot* (Ling Shu, 灵枢) of two thousands years ago, the earliest extant medical classics in China. *Plain Questions •The Art of Life Through the Four Seasons* (Su Wen • Siqi Tiaoshen Dalun, 素问•四气调神大论) states that "Therefore, the sages treat disease by preventing illness before it begins, just as a good government or emperor is able to take the necessary steps to avert war. Treating an illness after it has begun is like suppressing revolt after it has broken out. If someone digs a well when thirsty, or forges weapons after becoming engaged in battle, one cannot help but ask: Are not these actions too late?" *Miraculous Pivot • Counterflow and Smooth Flow* (Ling Shu • Ni Cong, 灵枢•逆顺) states that "A superior practitioner gives acupuncture treatment when the disease is not yet born. A secondary technique is to needle when it is not yet abundant. ... The superior prevents disease from occurring but does not treat what is already diseased. This is the saying". The above quotations show a pithy insight into the medical function of preventive treatment. Such an idea is discussed in *The Classic of Difficult Issues* (Nan Jing, 难经) and *Synopsis of the Golden Chamber* (Jinkui Yaolue, 金匮要略) of the Eastern Han Dynasty (25-220A.D.) and other works on Chinese medicine of all the ages after that, and has been continuously developed and perfected up till today.

The idea of "Preventive Treatment" in Chinese medicine can be summarized as "Three Preventions", namely "Preventing Illness from Occurring", "Preventing Illness from Progressing", and "Preventing Illness from Recurring".

1.1 Preventing Illness from Occurring

The idea of "Preventing Illness from Occurring", which is discussed in most of the Chinese medical classics, can be illustrated from the following two aspects, i.e., cultivating the internal healthy qi and avoiding the external pathogenic qi.

1.1.1 Cultivating the Internal Healthy Qi

The occurrence and development of a disease depend on the struggle between the healthy qi and the pathogenic qi. Generally speaking, the pathogenic qi cannot find the way to invade the body if the healthy qi takes a dominant role. That is to say, the body has strong body resistance. But it will be attacked by the pathogenic qi if the healthy qi is insufficient. Well then how to strengthen healthy qi? The ancients have shown the quiet and the moving ways to cultivate the healthy qi for the later generations.

In the quiet way, firstly, one should cultivate the mind. In the chapter *On the True Qi Endowed by Heaven in Remote Antiquity* of *Plain Questions* (Su Wen • Shanggu Tianzhen Lun, 素问 • 上古天真论) it states that "One should be indifferent to fame or gain or anything else in order to keep the true qi flowing smoothly and freely and maintain the spirit staying inside the body. Then where does illness come from"？, and that "The ancient people who understood the way of cultivating health followed the law of yin-yang of the four seasons, harmonized their bodies with the environment, took proper diets, and had a regular lifestyle. Thus, they did not show conventional signs of aging, and were able to keep the body and the mind united, thus could live beyond biological limitations until 100 years old"? With quiet, self-adaptive state of mind, the three treasures, essence, qi and spirit, stick to the body, so that it can not be encroached upon by any illness. Secondly, one should cultivate the body. The body and spirit coincide with each other through following the four seasons, yin and yang, proper diet and regular lifestyle without over consuming physical strength, so he is able to live beyond the natural life-span. This is healthy qi cultivation by the quiet way.

In the moving way, the physiological function of the body can be strengthened by moderate exercises, which promote the circulation of essence, qi, and blood, thus reinforcing the body resistance. *Lu's Spring and Autumn Annals • Jin Shu* (Lushi Chunqiu, 吕氏春秋• 尽数) states that "Running water is never stale and a door-hinge never gets worm-eaten because both are moving. This is indeed the case for the body and qi. If the body does not move, the essence will stop flowing, then qi stagnation will ensue". Therefore, our ancestors created a variety of exercises to keep fit. The famous regimen recorded in *Chuang Tzu • Deliberately* (Zhuang Zi • Keyi, 庄子 • 刻意) reads exhaling the turbid air and inhaling the clear with one's body shaped like a bear climbing a tree or a bird stretching its neck. According to the record in *History of the Later Han Dynasty • Divination* (Houhanshu • Fangshu Liezhuan, 后汉书 • 方术列传), Hua Tuo (华佗), a famous medical expert in Eastern Han Dynasty (25 - 220A.D.), developed a set of simple health gymnastics, "the five-animal exercises", which enhances body constitution by imitating the movement of the tiger, deer, bear, ape and bird. This is healthy qi cultivation by the moving way.

*Synopsis of the Golden Chamber* (Jinkui Yaolue, 金匮要略) points out in the chapter *On Pulse, Symptom **C**omplex and Transmission of Diseases of the Viscera, Bowels, Channels and Collaterals* (Zangfu Jingluo Xianhou Bing Mai Zheng, 藏府经络先后病脉证) that "One should carefully protect one's body resistance and avoid the attack of climatic pathogenic factors. Otherwise, Channels and Collaterals will have violated and health endangered". The above-mentioned two ways are the very basic measures "to carefully protect one's body resistance".

1.1.2 Avoiding External Pathogenic Qi

*Plain Questions* (Su Wen, 素问) and *Miraculous Pivot* (Ling Shu, 灵枢) never ignore the role of external pathogenic factors with the emphasis on the leading role of healthy qi in the occurrence and development of an illness. The chapter *On Needling Techniques* of *Plain Questions* (Su Wen • Cifa Lun, 素问•刺法论) warns people "to avoid toxic qi" after stating "The evil qi cannot find a way to invade the body if the healthy qi resides inside the body". *Miraculous Pivot* (Ling Shu, 灵枢) also points out that "The sages said that one should carefully avoid evils (or pathogenic factors) just like avoiding arrows and stones, then the evils cannot injure the body". "To avoid toxic qi" and "to avoid the evils" in the above mentioned quotations all exhort the people to take timely precautions to protect the body against severe pathogenic factors, including pollution sources by ecological destruction and various factors leading to iatrogenic and drug –induced diseases, just like to be against sharp arrows and hard stones.

1.2 Preventing Illness from Progressing

After the occurrence of a disease, one should understand its cause and mechanism, master the progressing rules of the disease from the exterior to the interior, from the superficial to the deep, and from the simple to the complicated, and then can strive for the therapeutic initiative. This idea contains the following three aspects:

### 1.2.1 Adopting Early Treatment

This idea emphasizes that during the treatment patients should be early diagnosed and treated in time based on the rules of occurrence and development of a disease, hence obstructing its development. In the chapter *On Images Corresponding to Yin-Yang* of *Plain Questions* (Su Wen • Yinyang Yingxiang Dalun, 素问• 阴阳应象大论) it states that "When the evil wind attacks people, it comes like a storm. We can map out its course of attack, beginning with the pores and skin, into the muscle layer, through the tendomuscular layer, into the vessels, and into the five zang and six fu organs. A superior doctor arrests disease at the skin level and dispels it before it penetrates deeper. An inferior doctor treats illness after it passes the skin. If the pathogen is not stopped on the surface, it enters the muscle level and must be dispersed there. If it progresses and invades deep into the five zang organs, the prognosis for recovery is only fifty percent". *Synopsis of the Golden Chamber* (Jinkui Yaolue, 金匮要略) also points out in the chapter *On Pulse, Symptom* ***C****omplex and Transmission of Diseases of the Viscera. Bowels, Channels and Collaterals* (Zangfu Jingluo Xianhou Bing Mai Zheng, 藏府经络先后病脉证) that "If there is heaviness and uneasiness in the extremities, Daoyin (Breathing and physical exercise therapy used in ancient times, similar to present-day *Qigong* therapy), Tuna (Breathing therapy practiced in ancient times), acupuncture and Gaomo (Rubbing areas affected with rheumatic or skin diseases with ointment) therapies should he practiced to clear the nine orifices". *Records of History • The Biography of Bianque and Canggong* (Shi Ji • Bianque Canggong Liezhuan, 史记 • 扁鹊仓公列传) states that "If the disease is in the striated layer of the skin, I can cure it with decoction and hot compression; in the blood vessels, with needles and medical stones; in the intestines and stomach, with medicinal wine; but in the bone marrow, nothing could be done even by the Life God!", and that "If wise people can know about their illness at an earlier stage and if superior doctors can give timely treatment, then the illnesses will be surely cured and life will be certainly ensured". All of these are aimed to indicate that the effective measures should be taken at the early stage of a disease when the pathogen stays in the skin and hair, the muscular interstice or the four limbs, otherwise the disease will worsen, then going deep into the bone marrow and the nine orifices will be obstructed. Then, no one is able to help under this condition even if he is as highly skilled as Bianque or authorized by the Life God.

1.2.2 Preventing Illness from Progressing and Changing

This idea stresses that in the process of treatment, the patients should be diagnosed and treated as soon as possible on the basis of progressing and changing routes of an illness, therefore stopping its progressing and changing. *The Classic of Difficult Issues • The 77th Issue* (Nan Jing, 难经 • 七十七难) reads that "The so-called preventive treatment implies the following: When one sees an illness in the liver, one should know that the liver will transmit it to the spleen. Hence one prevents this transmission by fortifying the spleen qi, with the effect that it will not be affected by the evil (pathogen) from the liver. Hence the scripture speaks of 'preventive treating'. When a mediocre practitioner sees an illness in the liver, he does not know about mutual transmission, and he will focus all his efforts on treating the liver. Hence the scripture speaks of his 'treating what is ill already'." According to the theory of the restraining relationship among the five phases, the liver disease tends to transfer to the spleen and stomach. Therefore, the application of strengthening the spleen and stomach when treating the liver disease is a preventive treatment which will stop such a development. This thinking and its applications were also used by Zhang Zhongjing (张仲景) in the chapter *On Pulse, Symptom Complex and Transmission of Diseases of the Viscera, Bowels, Channels and Collaterals* (Zangfu Jingluo Xianhou Bing Mai Zheng, 藏府经络先后病脉证) of *Synopsis of the Golden Chamber* (Jinkui Yaolue, 金匮要略) and still have important significance in the clinical practice up till today. Many practitioners of the later generations such as Xu Dachun (徐大椿), Ye Gui（叶桂）, et al continued to apply and develop such an idea, which are illustrated in their works such as the chapter *On Exterior & Interior, Upper & Lower* of *The Origin and Development of Chinese Medicine* (Yixue Yuanliu Lun • Biaoli Shangxia Lun, 医学源流论•表里上下论) and the chapter *Transmission to Ying-Nutrient Phase* of *Treatise on Warm and Febrile Diseases* (Wenre Lun • Dichuan Ruying, 温热论•递传入营)

1.2.3 Treating the External Manifestations of Illness

On the basis of Chinese medical theory – speculating internal pathological changes by observing the external appearance of life, pathological changes will reflect on the superficial of the body, so that illnesses can be early diagnosed and treated accordingly. In the chapter *On Protecting Life and Preserving Physical Appearance* of *Plain Questions* (Su Wen •

Baoming Quanxing Lun, 素问 • 保命全形论) it reads that "Salt stored in a container gradually seeps a fluid. This is the qi of the salt draining. A string on an instrument, on the verge of breaking, will display a brittle, high-pitched dying sound. A tree with shallow roots, although its branches and leaves are abundant, eventually will wither because its inside is empty. Certainly, when humans manifest conditions similar to these, we are told of severe damage to the internal organs. Because the skin, flesh, qi, and blood have become damaged and drained, it will be difficult to rejuvenate the person, even with the intervention of acupuncture, herbs, and moxibustion". In the chapter *On Needling Febrile Diseases* of *Plain Questions* (Su Wen • Cire Lun, 素问 • 刺热论), even the pathological changes of febrile diseases of the internal five zang organs may be detected by the outside manifestation of red face. This is preventive treatment that the patients should be treated in time before the outbreak of a disease.

1.3 Preventing Illness from Recurring

During the rehabilitation phase when the healthy qi hasn't regained its strength, abstinence and regimen are typically important for people to prevent the disease from recurring. Ancient Chinese medical classics hold that reasons for recurrence mainly involve improper diet, over work and excessive sexual intercourse. For example, *General Treatise on Causes and Manifestations of All Diseases* (Zhubing Yuanhou Lun, 诸病源候论) discusses various kinds of recurrences induced by diet, work, sexual intercourse as well as too much thinking and talking in many chapters. As regards to food-induced recurrence by improper diet, it is especially extensively discussed in the ancient Chinese medical literature. For example, in the chapter *On Febrile Diseases* of *Plain Questions* (Su Wen • Re Lun, 素问•热论), it states that "When such patients are fed animal products that are difficult to digest, the disease will recur. If they eat large quantities, too, this will cause more accumulation. Therefore, overeating or taking in animal products should be avoided during febrile disease.", and that "In general, patients have residual heat because they were force-fed food during the severe part of febrile diseases. The heat subsequently cannot be completely cleared. The pathogen must be cleared before much eating is done; otherwise food will be undigested and cause more heat." If this aims at preventing febrile diseases from recurring from improper diets, *Plain Question • Rules of Phase Energetics* (Su Wen •Wu Changzheng Dalun,

素问•五常政大论) expounds the significance of building up health by using medicine and taking nourishing food, "Specifically, when administering medicine, once the health is sixty percent recovered, withdraw the extreme toxic medicinals; once the health is seventy percent recovered, withdraw the moderate toxic medicinals; once the health is eighty percent recovered, withdraw the mildly toxic medicinals; once the health is ninety percent recovered, withdraw the nontoxic medicinals. Follow up with special food, herbs and dietetic remedies for regeneration. Following this principle, a physician will be successful in patients' care."

2. Cultural Connotations of Preventive Treatment

The concept of culture can be understood in the broad and narrow senses. In a broad sense, culture refers to the accumulation of substantial and spiritual wealth created in the practice of human society along the history; in a narrow sense, culture means ideology in a society. The philosophy of preventive treatment originates from the awareness of hardship of the Chinese nation. This awareness has a time-honored history in China since its formation as early as in Yin and Zhou Dynasties (C.1600-221 B.C.). After the overthrow of the reign of Yin (C.1600-C.1100 B.C.), King Wu of Zhou Dynasty (Zhou Wu Wang, 周武王), deeply reflected on the lessons of Xia Jie [夏桀, the last king of Xia Dynasty (C.2100-C.1600 B.C.)] and Yin Zhou [殷纣, the last king of Shang Dynasty (C.1600-C.1100 B.C.)], who became the last governors of their reigns in stead of being exalted, and realized the laws of leading to qualitative change from quantitative change just like "failing to build a high mountain for want of one final basket of soil", so that he kept a strong awareness of hardship. From the 11$^{th}$ century B.C. until the 3$^{rd}$ century B.C., the Zhou Dynasty had lasted for eight hundred years, so far becoming the dynasty under the longest reign in the Chinese history.

The awareness of hardship not only refers to understanding the hardships in the reality or foretelling the possible hardships in the future, and the more important is to remove those which have already appeared and to prevent the possible ones from occurring. Awareness of hardship, as a kind of man's awareness, is not only the subject's initiative real reaction to the passive object, but also acts as the subject's guide in directing object to "give up vice and return to virtue", which is actually the collective reflection of the man's wisdom, boldness and resolution. The hardship in "the awareness of hardship" is realistic, or could be realistic, therefore is radically different from "the case of a man of Qi feared that the sky might fall" (杞人忧天) – here I mean "the groundless fears" or "making trouble out of nothing".

The relationship between the awareness of hardship and preventive treatment can be discussed in the following two aspects.

2.1 Thinking of Danger in Times of Safety

"Thinking of danger in times of safety" is extensively discussed in the oldest extant Confucian classics in China, such as *The Book of Songs* (Shi Jing, 诗经), *The Book of Documents* (Shang Shu, 尚书), and *The Book of Changes* (Yi Jing, 易经). *The Book of Songs* records that before raining, the strigidae have started to nest, wrapping their door by the roots and barks peeled off from the mulberry trees. The idiom "Wei Yu Chou Mou 未雨绸缪 - repair the nest (house) before it rains" comes from this story. Bo Yi (伯益), the minister in Yao (尧) and Shun (舜) period in the remote antiquity, a grand senior man, said to Da Yu (大禹): "Ah! You should be cautious! I keep on warning you against lawlessness, indulgence and over enjoyment", which implicates if Da Yu doesn't take his advice, the country will be subjugated. It shows BoYi's expression for his awareness of thinking of danger in times of safety. *The Book of Changes*, sprouting in Yin (殷) and Zhou (周) period, is a divination book for foretelling good or bad fortunes by using shi （蓍） grass, as well as a philosophical literature full of such an awareness of hardship. It states that "Does the author who composed *The I* (referring to *The Book of Changes*) not have the awareness of hardship?" This is an overall portrayal of the entire book.

Confucius comments the PI or Hindrance (否) that "Forget not! Forget not! Tying up the trunks of mulberry trees". "Baosang" in this quotation refers to the trunks of mulberry trees. This saying means things that are tied to the trunk stays very firm. It is further explained this in the name of Confucius that the danger happens because it is thought the past prosperity can be lasting, so that it is felt dauntless about prosperity, resulting in present misery; an ending disaster happens because it is thought that the past being can be eternal, and therefore felt fearless, leading to today's extinction; the misfortune happens because it is thought the past peace can be going on forever, and hence felt careless, thus causing today's catastrophe. Thus a man of honor in prosperity must not forget danger at every moment, and always worries if he will be wiped out, firmly linking his safety to the trunks of mulberry trees.

Is the "preventive treatment" in Chinese medicine really indeed the case? Present illness is due to his thought that the past health can be lasting and he feels careless and no fears about his health, thus leading to today's critical disease. Therefore, in health, it is very necessary to prevent the pathogenic factors from invading the body all the time. *Lao Tzu* states in its 71st chapter that "Who recognizes his limitations is healthy; Who ignores his limitations is sick. The sage recognizes this sickness as a limitation. And so becomes immune". Just from the perspective on disease, Lao Tzu taught us that only if we treat carefully the possible disease should we enjoy health. On the contrary, if we don't treat carefully the possible disease, we can't keep fit, which is surely the behavior of the inferior.

Let's probe into the matter. As regards to the time of the hardship, the real hardship does not lie in the time of being hardship, but its very opposite – the time of being peaceful and happy; The real hardship does not exist in the person with the hardship, but exist in the person with peace and happiness. The time of being satisfied with the peace is just the time of being shrouded by a certain hardship; the person who enjoys his happiness will surely become the carrier of hardship. It is also stated in *The Book of Songs* that one should be trembling with fears, i.e. should be very cautious as if he is standing upon the edge of an abyss or treading on eggs; for people who is not in such a situation, he should also be cautious as if he is in a real situation.

Is the "preventive treatment" in Chinese medicine not the same as "the awareness of hardship" stated here? The real hardship does not occur after being diseased, but happens to its very opposite – the time before an illness begins; the real hardship does not exist in the persons with illnesses, but exists in those without illnesses. Real concern doesn't come up after falling ill, but just its very opposite, before falling ill. Once he is in a walking-on-eggs situation or falling ill, he should have optimism to take things as they come and summon up his will to face danger without fear, actively cooperating with the doctor so that he is able to apply medical techniques to relieve the situation.

The awareness of hardship is also expounded thoroughly in *Mencius* (孟子)- Without expostulations from loyal ministers at home and challenges from other enemy countries, the country will inevitably die, therefore from which the truth is revealed that one thrives in calamity and perishes in soft living. There is a phenomenon called "Catfish Effect": A few catfishes that eat small fishes are put into the fish tank in order to keep the sardines alive to the port before they are made into cans. The catfishes drive the sardines running all around and thus they can get enough oxygen which keeps them alive to the port. The "Catfish Effect" shows that crisis can inspire energy, which just confirms the universal significance of the truth that "one thrives in calamity and perishes in soft living".

You will be safe if you think of danger in times of safety, while you will be in danger if you think of safety in times of safety; You will stay in a healthy state if you think of preventive measures before illnesses begin, while you will get ill if you do not take preventive measures to prevent illnesses from occurring. That is where the relationship between the awareness of hardship (i.e. thinking of danger in times of safety) and "preventive treatment" lies in.

### 2.2 Nipping An Evil in the Bud

Nipping An Evil in the Bud – putting an end to something while it is in the beginning stage, an awareness of hardship, is based on the differentiation between good or bad fortunes and measurement of changes from quantity to quality.

As the above mentioned, *The Book of Changes* is a divination book for foretelling good or bad fortunes. Thus, by using the three hundred and eighty six yao (爻), this book tells people again and again what are bad fortunes, what are good ones, how to avoid bad ones and how to tend towards good ones. In the 58th chapter of *Lao Tzu* it states that "Good fortune follows upon disaster; Disaster lurks within good fortune; Who can say how things will end? Perhaps there is no end. Honesty is ever deceived; Kindness is ever seduced; Men have been like this for a long time. So the sage is firm but not cutting, pointed but not piercing, straight but not rigid, bright but not blinding."*Lao Tzu* holds that contradictions like weal and woe, the positive and negative, the good and evil coexist together in a unity, depending on each other and transforming into each other without end, which embodies the rule of inter-dependence and inter-transformation between them. *Lao Tzu* asks people to pay attention to the information of changes between the good and bad fortunes, so as to tend towards good ones and avoid bad ones.

As regards to the process from qualitative change to quantitative change, it originates from the 64th chapter of *Lao Tzu*: "What lies still is easy to grasp; What lies far off is easy to anticipate; What is brittle is easy to shatter; What is small is easy to disperse. Yet a tree broader than a man can embrace is born of a tiny shoot; A dam greater than a river can overflow starts with a clod of earth; A journey of a thousand miles begins at the spot under one's feet. Therefore deal with things before they happen; Create order before there is confusion." It shows that things develop along the rules from the small to the big, the tiny to the huge, the quantitative to the qualitative. Badness such as regicide and patricide does not happen in a day but is developed with an inevitable trend like from frost to ice. In order to prevent things from transforming to the bad side, it is necessary to be conscious of its source at the beginning. This is what we say from the first small beginnings one can see how things will develop.

Confucius comments the Kun or Responding (坤) that " The family that heaps goodness upon goodness is sure to have an abundance of blessings. The family that piles evil upon evil is sure to have an abundance of misery. Murder of a ruler by his minister, or a father by his son, does not result from a single day and night? Its causes have accumulated bit by bit through the absence of early discrimination. *The Book of Changes* says, 'Treading on hoarfrost, solid ice will come.' It shows the natural sequence of cause and effect."

Therefore, the ancient Chinese philosophers attached vital importance to "Jian Ji" (见几) stated in *The Book of Changes*, i.e. putting an end to sth. while it is in the beginning stage, nipping an evil in the bud, which is really indeed the same as the meanings of some statements in ancient Chinese medical classics, such as "A superior doctor arrests disease at the skin level and dispels it before it penetrates deeper. An inferior doctor treats illness after it passes the skin. If the pathogen is not stopped on the surface, it enters the muscle level and must be dispersed there. If it progresses and invades deep into the five zang organs, the prognosis for recovery is only fifty percent" from the chapter *On Images Corresponding to Yin-Yang* of *Plain Questions* (Su Wen • Yinyang Yingxiang Dalun, 素问• 阴阳应象大论). Besides, "Preventive Treatment" was also the yardstick to evaluate the levels of practitioners of Chinese medicine in ancient China.

*Huai-nan Tzu* (淮南子) states in the chapter of *Discourse on Mountains* (说山训) that "A superior doctor always adopts treatment to prevent illnesses from occurring; A sage often takes measures to avoid hardship from happening.", which demonstrates the common ground shared by "preventive treatment" in Chinese medicine and "awareness of hardship" in Chinese culture.

Junpeng Gao and Dingfang Cai

# Triptolide protects against 1-methyl-4-phenyl pyridinium ($MPP^+$)-induced dopaminergic neurotoxicity in rats: Implication for immunosuppressive therapy in Parkinson's disease

*Objective*: Neuroinflammation with microglial activation has been implicated to have a strong association with the progressive dopaminergic neuronal loss in Parkinson's disease (PD). The present study was undertaken to evaluate the activation profile of microglia in 1-methyl-4-phenyl pyridinium ($MPP^+$)-induced hemiparkinsonian rats. Triptolide, a potent immunosuppressant and microglia inhibitor, was then examined for its efficacy in protecting dopaminergic neurons from injury and ameliorating behavioral disabilities induced by $MPP^+$. *Methods*: The rat model of PD was established by intranigral microinjection of $MPP^+$. At baseline and on d 1, 3, 7, 14, 21 following $MPP^+$ injection, the degree of microglial activation was examined by detecting the immunodensity of OX-42 (microglia marker) in the substantia nigra (SN). The number of viable dopaminergic neurons was determined by measuring tyrosine hydroxylase (TH) positive neurons in the SN. Behavioral performances were evaluated by counting the number of rotations induced by, apomorphine calculating scores of forelimb akinesia and vibrissae-elicited forelimb placing asymmetry. *Results*: Intranigral injection of $MPP^+$ resulted in robust activation of microglia, progressive depletion of dopaminergic neurons, and ongoing aggravation of behavioral disabilities in rats. Triptolide significantly inhibited microglial activation, partially prevented dopaminergic cells from death and improved behavioral performances. *Conclusion*: These data demonstrated for the first time a neuroprotective effect of triptolide on dopaminergic neurons in $MPP^+$-induced hemiparkinsonian rats. The protective effect of triptolide may, at least partially, be related to the inhibition of $MPP^+$-induced microglial activation. Our results lend strong support to the use of immunosuppressive agents in the management of PD.

## 1. Introduction

Parkinson's disease (PD) is one of the most common age-related neurodegenerative diseases[1]. Clinically, most patients suffer from slowness of movement, rest tremor, rigidity, and disturbances in balance. Pathologically, it is characterized by the progressive degeneration of dopaminergic neurons in the substantia nigra (SN)[2,3]. Although symptomatic treatments of PD are of proven efficacy, no drug has been established to have a clinically validated effect on slowing down its progression[4,5]. Better understanding of these processes leading to progressive dopaminergic neuronal loss may provide effective targets for the design of novel therapeutics to PD.

Neuroinflammation have currently been implicated as a driving force in PD pathogenesis[6]. Microglia are suspected to play a major role in this process. As constitutive immune cells in the brain, microglia are sensitive to even minor disturbances in central nervous system (CNS) homeostasis and become readily activated in response to abnormal stimulation[7]. Uncontrolled activation of microglia may cause direct toxicity to neurons by releasing various cytotoxic compounds[8]. Activated microglia have been found not only in post-mortem PD brain, but also in various PD models[9-11]. Inhibition of microglia-mediated neuroinflammation, therefore, might become a promising therapeutic strategy in PD[12].

We focused on triptolide, an active component derived from the traditional Chinese medicinal plant *Tripterygium Wilfordii* Hook F (TWHF), which has anti-inflammatory and immunosuppressive activities[13,14,15]. In the CNS, triptolide is capable of blocking lipopolysaccharide (LPS)-induced activation of microglia[16,17]. However, whether triptolide could inhibit microglial activation and exert neuroprotective effect in 1-methyl-4-phenyl pyridinium ($MPP^+$)-induced hemiparkinsonian rats still remain unknown.

The aim of the present study was, first, to evaluate the activation profile of microglia in $MPP^+$-induced hemiparkinsonian rats, an ideal animal model of PD[18]. Then, we sought to investigate the effect of triptolide on microglial activation, and examined whether it could exert neuroprotective effect against $MPP^+$ neurotoxicity.

## 2. Materials and methods

### 2.1 Animals

Experiments were performed on adult male Sprague-Dawley rats (Experimental Animal Center, Shanghai Medical College of Fudan University, China) weighing 250-280 g. Rats were housed in suspended cages and maintained on a 12:12 h light-dark cycle with free access to food and water. All experimental protocols and animal handling procedures were approved by Animal Care and Use Committee (ACUC) of Fudan University, and were consistent with the National Institutes of Healthy Guide for the Care and Use of laboratory animals. All efforts were made to minimize the number of animals used and their suffering.

### 2.2 Intranigral injection of $MPP^+$

Before surgery, 54 rats were randomly divided into nine groups (6 animals each). Six groups received $MPP^+$ alone and were subjected to behavioral and immunohistochemical analysis at baseline (d 0) and on d 1, 3, 7, 14, 21 after surgery. One group received saline instead of $MPP^+$ and served as sham control. The remaining two groups were treated by intraperitoneal (i.p.) injection of triptolide and normal saline (NS) respectively following $MPP^+$ injection. During surgery, all animals were securely placed into a sterotaxic device (Jiangwan, Shanghai, China) under Chloral Hydrate (400 mg/kg, i.p.) anesthesia with bregma and lambda at a horizontal level. All stereotaxic coordinates were determined according to the brain atlas of Paxinos and Watson[19]. For intranigral microinjection, a small hole was drilled in the skull above the left SN (5.0 mm anteroposterior, 2.1 mm lateral). A microsyringe was then lowered (7.7 mm dorsoventral), and 10 μg of $MPP^+$ (Sigma, USA) (5 μg/μL) in a saline buffer was infused at a rate of 0.4 μL/min for 5 min. After infusion of the toxin, the probe was kept in the same position for a further 5 min for complete diffusion of the drug and then slowly retracted. The post-operative animals were left in a temperature-controlled chamber until they recovered from anesthesia, then they returned to their home cage.

### 2.3 Administration of drugs

Triptolide (purity: 98%) was provided by National Institute for the Control of Pharmaceutical and Biological Products (No. 111567-200502). Administration of triptolide was principally consistent with the method described previously[17]. Briefly, triptolide was dissolved in saline containing 5% dimethylsulphoxide and applied intraperitoneally. Rats received a single dose of 5 µg/kg triptolide or vehicle per day from 3 d before $MPP^+$ injection and continued for 21 d post-lesion (24 d in total).

2.4 Behavioral tests

The degree of damage to nigrostriatal pathway can be assessed using sensitive drug and non-drug tests. A series of tests was performed before and on d 1, 3, 7, 14 and 21 after surgery.

2.4.1 Rotational behavior analysis:

At all the above mentioned time points, rats were injected subcutaneously with 0.3 mg/kg apomorphine hydrochloride (Sigma, USA) dissolved in 0.1% ascorbate saline solution and allowed to sit in a separate cage for 15 min. Animals were then placed in an iron bowl, and the net number of turns (made towards the side of lesion minus those made away from the lesioned side) in a 30-min trial was calculated[20].

2.4.2 Forelimb akinesia (stepping test)

Movement initiation for each limb was assessed using the forelimb akinesia test protocol[21-23]. In short, the rat was hold by the experimenter with one hand fixing the hindlimbs and slightly raising the hind part above the surface. The animal was allowed to initiate stepping movements in a 10 sec period for the left forelimb and then the right one for a balanced order. An ipsilateral asymmetry score was derived [(ipsilteral steps/ipsilateral plus contralateral steps) - (contralateral steps/ipsilateral plus contralateral steps)].

2.4.3 Vibrissae-elicited forelimb placing

A vibrissae-elicited forelimb-placing test was used to test reaction to sensory stimuli as described previously[22-25]. At the assigned time points after surgery, rats were gently held by their torsos with the forelimbs hung free. The respective vibrissae of the animal were brushed against the corner edge of a countertop to elicit a forelimb placing response from the forelimb on the same side. Intact animals place the forelimb of both sides quickly onto the countertop. Animals with unilateral damage will show varying degrees of impaired limb placing ability, while still placing the unimpaired limb reliably. Each animal was tested 10 times on each side. Percentage of unsuccessful placing responses was determined [(number placed contralaterally divided by the number placed ipsilaterally)×10].

2.5 Immunohistochemistry and quantification

As previously described by our group[26], rats were given an overdose of urethane (2 g/kg, i.p.) and perfused intracardially with 100 mL 0.9% saline followed by 400 mL cold 4% paraformaldehyde in 0.1 mol/L phosphate buffer (PB, pH 7.4). Brains were removed and immersed from 10%-30% gradient sucrose in PB for 24-48 h at 4 °C for cryoprotection. Coronal brain sections (free-floating, 30 μm) were cut by a freezing microtome (Leica 1900, German) and processed for immunofluorescence. All the sections were blocked with 10% normal donkey serum in 0.01 mol/L phosphate buffered saline (PBS, pH 7.4) with 0.3% Triton-X-100 for 1 h at room temperature and incubated over night at 4 °C with mouse anti-OX-42 (1:1000, Sigma, USA), rabbit anti-tyrosine hydroxylase (TH) (1:1000, Sigma, USA) primary antibody. The sections were then incubated with fluorescein isothiocyanate (FITC)-conjugated donkey anti-mouse IgG (1:200, Chemicon, USA) or rhodamine-conjugated donkey anti-rabbit IgG (1:200, Chemicon, USA) for 90 min at 4 °C, then washed in PBS. Omission of primary antibody served as negative control. The stained sections were examined with a Leica fluorescence microscope, and images were captured with a CCD spot camera.

Because the morphology of microglia is complex and the immunoreactive staining includes both cell bodies and their processes, cell counts may not sufficiently quantify activation. Therefore, the integrated densities (pixelwise integration of density) of OX-42 immunoreactivity (OX-42-IR) within the SN were measured with the Leica Qwin 500 image analysis system (Germany) at six randomly selected sections for each animal.

Quantification of viable dopaminergic neurons were principally consistent with a method previously descried by Vaananen, AJ *et al.* with slight modifications[27]. TH is the rate-limiting enzyme in the synthesis of catecholamines, and specific for catecholaminergic neurons. Thus, quantification of TH-positive neurons in serial sections throughout the SN can be used as a reliable measure for the numbers of viable dopaminergic neurons. The relative numbers of TH-positive neurons were evaluated by counting TH-positive neurons at six randomly selected sections within the SN area in both ipsilateral (injected) and contralateral (non-injected) side under the fluorescence microscope. The results were expressed as a percentage of TH-positive neurons at the injected side compared to the non-injected side, and the percentages for each experimental group were pooled.

2.6 Statistical analysis

Differences of immunohistochemical and behavioral data between two groups at a single time point were performed by student's *t*-test. One-way ANOVA followed by Holm-Sidak *t*-test was employed for analyzing percentage of TH-positive neurons and behavioral data at different time points after $MPP^+$ injection. Two-way ANOVA (treatment×time) followed by Newman–Keuls post hoc test was used for analyzing behavioral data between groups at different time points. Results have been presented as Mean ± SEM and $P < 0.05$ were considered significant.

2.7 Experimental procedure

2.7.1 Experiment 1: Effects of intranigral $MPP^+$ injection on microglial activation and TH-positive cell loss in rats

After baseline behavioral assessments, rats received intranigral injection of 10 µg/2 µL $MPP^+$. On d 0, 1, 3, 7, 14, and 21 after surgery, rats were perfused with fixative and the brains were removed for immunohistochemistry analysis. Quantification of the density of OX-42-IR and percentage of TH-positive neurons were performed as described in the previous section. The rats of sham group received an intranigral injection of sterile NS (2 µL) and were killed at d 21 after NS injection.

2.7.2 Experiment 2: Effects of $MPP^+$ on behavioral performances in rats

Behavioral performances were evaluated before sacrifice at different time points by performing forelimb akinesia, vibrissae-elicited forelimb placing and apomorphine induced rotation tests. Data in the $MPP^+$ group were compared with those in saline group.

2.7.3 Experiment 3: Effects of triptolide on $MPP^+$-induced microglial activation and TH-positive cell loss

After behavioral assessments on the d 21 post-surgery, rats were subjected to immunohistochemistry. The degree of microglial activation and TH-positive neuronal loss in the sham group, $MPP^+$ group, triptolide treatment group, and vehicle treatment group was examined by detecting OX-42-IR density and the percentage of TH-positive neuronal number ipsilateral to the $MPP^+$ injected side compared to the contralateral side.

2.7.4 Experiment 4: Effects of triptolide on $MPP^+$-induced behavioral defects in rats

Behavioral abnormalities of rats from all the experimental groups were examined at different time points after $MPP^+$ intoxication. Items of testing were the same as the behavioral tests described previously.

## 3. Results

### 3.1 Intranigrally injected $MPP^+$ induced microglial activation and dopaminergic neuronal loss in the SN area of rats

Activated microglia have been implicated in PD[10,28]. In order to examine the time course of microglial activation during the 21 d after $MPP^+$ injection, brain sections were immunostained with an antibody at different time points against OX-42 (CD-11b), a marker of activated microglia. In control animals, OX-42-immunopositive microglia in the intact SN exhibited the characteristics of inactive, resting microglia, and possessed small cell bodies. In rats treated with $MPP^+$, however, there was a marked increase in the number of OX-42-immunopositive microglia with morphological changes typical of activation. Activated microglia exhibited large cell bodies with multiple, thick and short lamellipodia (Fig. 1A), which was consistent with previous studies[29]. The density of OX-42-IR significantly increased at day 3 post-lesion ($t = 2.867$, $P < 0.05$), and reached the peak at d 7 ($t = 7.046$, $P < 0.05$). At d 14 and d 21 post-lesion, the increase in OX-42-IR became less marked ($t = 5.050$, $P < 0.05$; $t = 4.186$, $P < 0.05$; Fig. 1B).

Intranigral $MPP^+$ injection induced ongoing reduction of dopaminergic neurons as assessed by their expression of TH in SN ipsilateral to the $MPP^+$ injection site (Fig. 1C). The decrease in the percentage of TH-positive neurons became statistically significant at the third day post-lesion ($t = 3.731$, $P < 0.05$) and progressively manifested during the subsequent days of observation [One-way ANOVA, $F(5,30) = 81.453$, $P < 0.05$; Fig. 1D].

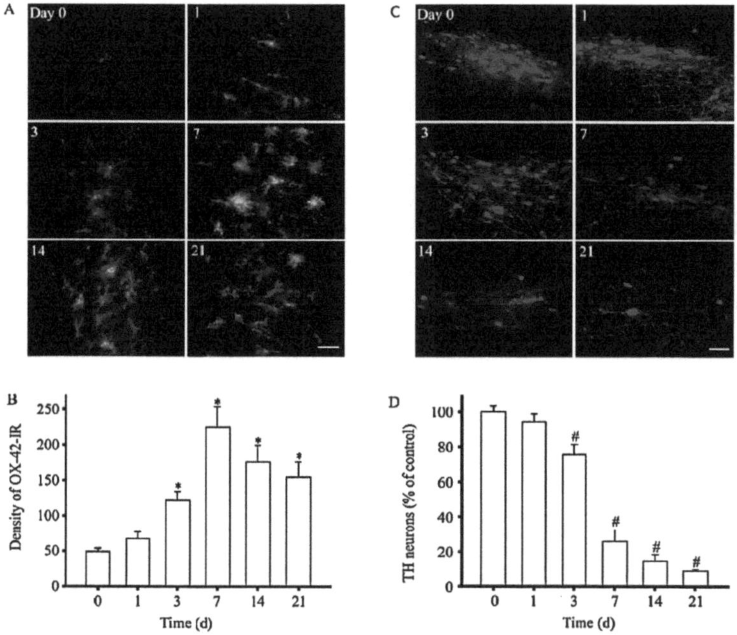


Fig. 1: Microglial cells and dopaminergic neurons in the SN as revealed with OX-42 and TH immunoreactivity respectively. A, Morphological presentation of OX-42-immunopositive microglia in the SN of rats at different time points after $MPP^+$ injection. Bar = 50 μm. B, Density of OX-42-IR in the SN of rats following intranigral $MPP^+$ injection. C, Representative photomicrographs showing TH immunopositivity in the SN of rats at different time points after $MPP^+$ injection. Bar = 100 μm. D, Quantification of the numbers of TH-positive neurons in the injected ipsilateral SN as compared with the contralateral non-injected SN, expressed as a percentage ratio. Data were represented as Mean±SEM. $^*P < 0.05$, $^\#P < 0.05$ *vs* baseline ($n = 6$).

## 3.2 Intranigrally injected $MPP^+$ induced progressive behavioral abnormalities in rats

Unilateral nigrostriatal lesions produce asymmetries in body posture and limb use in rats. Apomorphine induced rotational behavior, forelimb akinesia and vibrissae-elicited forelimb placing tests have been widely used in hemiparkinsonian rat model of PD as good indicators of damage to the nigrostriatal pathway[20,22,23,25,30]. Here, statistically significant behavioral defects occurred from the seventh day following intranigral $MPP^+$ injection (rotational behavior: $t = 5.485$, $P < 0.05$; forelimb akinesia: $t = 6.869$, $P <$

0.05; vibrissae-elicited forelimb placing: $t = 7.737$, $P < 0.05$). Such defects progressively worsened during the subsequent 14 d of observation [One-way ANOVA, rotational behavior: $F(2,15) = 20.441$, $P < 0.05$; forelimb akinesia: $F(2,15) = 11.141$, $P < 0.05$; vibrissae-elicited forelimb placing: $F(2,15) = 6.822$, $P < 0.05$; Fig. 2].

Our results are broadly in accordance with previous study by Banerjee R *et al.* who showed that intranigral $MPP^+$ infusion cause long-lasting damage to the nigrostriatal dopamine pathway, and did not show any sign of recovery in striatal dopamine content even after 90 d[31].

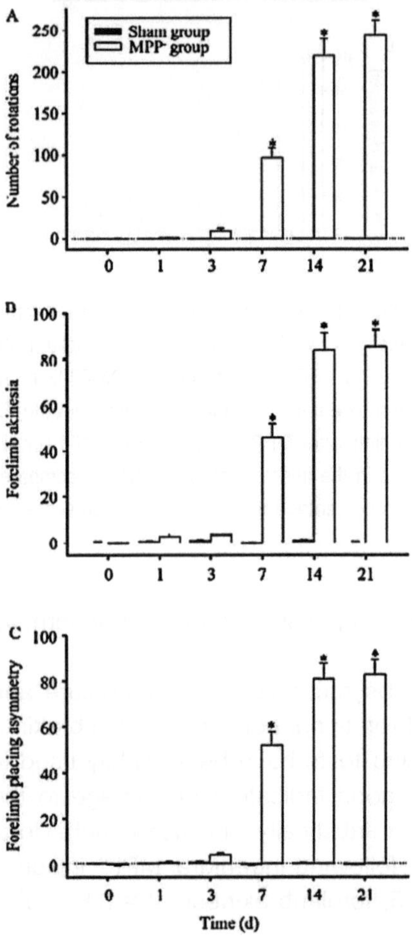


Fig. 2: Behavioral performances at different time points after MPP+ intoxication. Unilateral, 10 μg infusions of $MPP^+$ resulted in significant behavioral disabilities as assessed by apomorphine induced rotational behavior(A), forelimb akinesia(B), and vibrissae-elicited forelimb placing tests (C). Data were represented as Mean±SEM. $^*P < 0.05$ *vs* the control group ($n = 6$).

3.3 Triptolide attenuated $MPP^+$-induced microglial activation and dopaminergic neuronal loss

According to previous studies, triptolide is a potent anti-inflammatory and immunosuppressive agent, and is capable of inhibiting LPS-induced microglial activation and dopaminergic neuronal loss[13,16]. Here, we extended these studies to examine whether triptolide could quench $MPP^+$-induced microglial activation and protect dopaminergic cells from $MPP^+$ neurotoxicity.

While the $MPP^+$ group of rats exhibited increased OX-42-IR in the ipsilateral SN at 21 d post-lesion, the density of OX-42-IR in the triptolide treatment group were much attenuated and were statistically not different from the sham group ($t = 1.043$, $P = 0.304$), corroborating an inhibitory effect of triptolide on microglial activation (Fig. 3A, B).

The percentage of TH-positive neurons decreased in the SN ipsilateral to the $MPP^+$ injection site as compared with the contralateral side at 21 d post-lesion ($t = 11.008$, $P < 0.05$). Triptolide provided partially neuroprotection against dopaminergic neuronal loss as indicated by a much higher percentage of TH-positive neurons in the triptolide treatment group compared with the $MPP^+$ group ($t = 3.050$, $P < 0.05$) (Fig.3A, C). In the vehicle treatment group of rats, the density of OX-42-IR and the percentage of TH-positive neurons were principally not different from the $MPP^+$ group ($t = 0.078$, $P = 0.939$; $t = 0.421$, $P = 0.683$; Fig. 3B, C).

3.4 Triptolide mitigated behavioral abnormalities in $MPP^+$ intoxicated rats

Since triptolide was capable of preserving dopaminergic neurons from $MPP^+$-induced cell death, we then further our study to investigate whether triptolide could attenuate $MPP^+$-induced behavioral defects in rats.

As shown in previous sections, intranigral injection of $MPP^+$ resulted in progressive locomotor disabilities. In rats treated with triptolide, there was a noticeable attenuation of behavioral defects between 7 to 21 d (Fig. 4). Two-way ANOVA revealed significant effect of triptolide treatment (rotational behavior: $F(3,135) = 89.051$, $P < 0.05$; forelimb akinesia: $F(3,135) = 97.932$, $P < 0.05$; vibrissae-elicited forelimb placing: $F(3,135) = 105.091$ , $P < 0.05$) and interaction between triptolide treatment and time (rotational behavior: $F(3,135) = 21.902$, $P < 0.05$; forelimb akinesia: $F(3,135) = 20.798$, $P < 0.05$; vibrissae-elicited forelimb placing: $F(3,135) = 20.906$, $P < 0.05$).

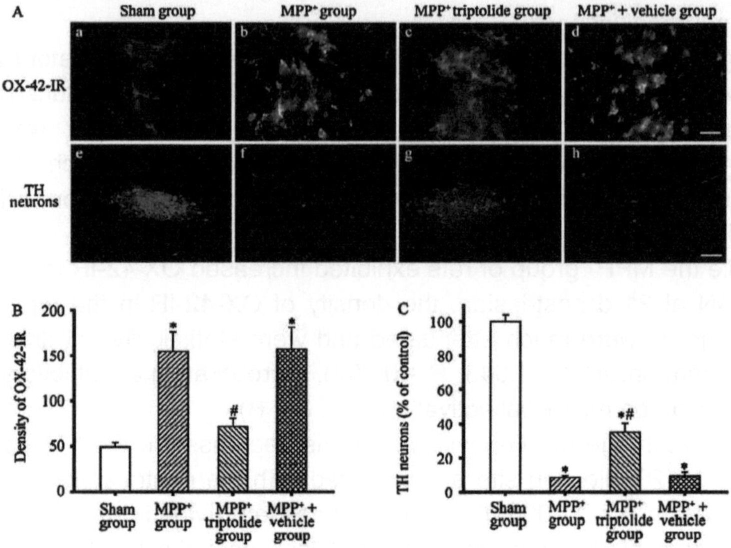


Fig. 3

Fig. 3: Effect of triptolide on MPP+-induced microglial activation and dopaminergic neurotoxicity in rats. A, Representative photomicrographs showing OX-42 (microglial marker) and TH (dopaminergic neuronal marker) in the injected SN area. OX-42 immunostaining in green (Aa, b, c, d), Bar = 50 μm; TH-positive neurons in red (Ae, f, g, h), Bar = 200 μm. B, Quantification of OX-42 immunoreactivity of different groups. Data were expressed as density of OX-42-IR. C, Quantification of the TH-positive neurons in the injected SN as compared to those in the contralateral non-injected SN, expressed as a percentage ratio. Data were represented as Mean±SEM. $^{*}P < 0.05$ *vs* sham group; $^{\#}P < 0.05$ *vs* $MPP^+$ group ($n = 6$).

Such results are consistent with the suggestion that anti-inflammatory and immunosuppressive agents are neuroprotective and may improve motor function in PD animals[32,33]. In the vehicle treated group, the behavioral defects were not ameliorated compared with the $MPP^+$ group at all the time points observed.

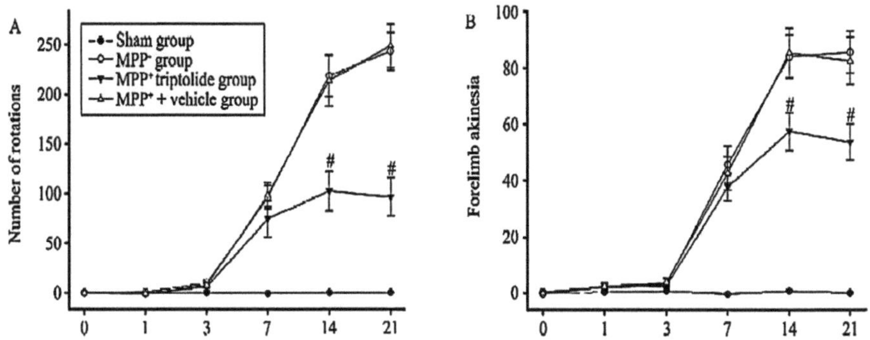


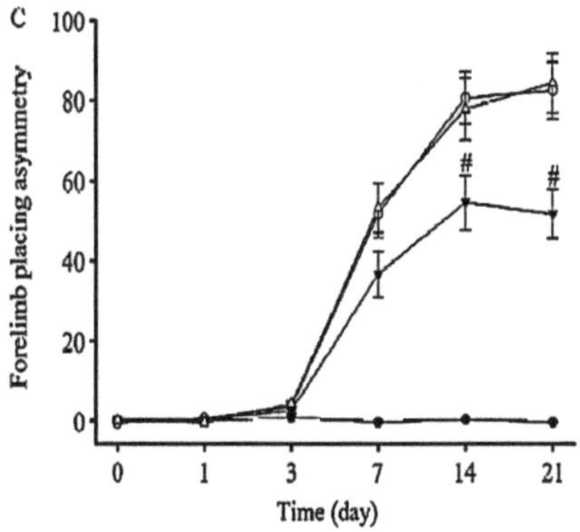


**Fig. 4** Effect of triptolide on MPP+-induced behavioral abnormalities in rats. While MPP+ led to progressive behavioral disabilities in rats, administration of triptolide resulted in attenuated locomotor defects as evaluated by apomorphine induced rotational behavior (A), forelimb akinesia (B), and vibrissae-elicited forelimb placing tests (C) between 7 to 21 d. Data were represented as Mean±SEM. #$P < 0.05$, *vs* the MPP+ group ($n = 6$).

## 4. Discussion

The search for neuroprotective agents in PD is primarily based on the ability of a specific drug to reduce dopaminergic neuronal loss. Agents that can provide such neuroprotective effects have the potential to become novel therapeutics to PD[4,5].

Existing animal models of PD provide us with useful tools to test new neuroprotective agents and strategies. 1-methyl-4-phenyl-1,2,3,6-tetrahydropyridine (MPTP) and its active metabolite, $MPP^+$, represent ideal neurotoxins that can replicates most features of sporadic PD in various animals[35]. However, if MPTP is systemically administered, not only dopaminergic neurons but also other cell types, particularly the glial cells will be affected simultaneously[29]. Because the enzymatic conversion of MPTP to $MPP^+$ by monoamine oxidase (MAO)-B mainly occurs in astrocyte[35-37], and drugs that can increase MAO activity have been shown to aggravate the neurotoxicity of MPTP by producing more $MPP^{+}$[29,36], therefore, study of neuroprotective agents using MPTP model of PD is open to multiple interpretations including the influence of astrocyte by the drugs tested. The $MPP^{+}$-induced hemiparkinsonian rats, thus, can be used as a reliable tool to understand the pathogenic relationships between microglial reaction and dopaminergic neurons, without having to concern about possible interference of astrocyte-neuron interaction. After $MPP^{+}$ enters into dopaminergic neurons through dopamine transporter (DAT), it is concentrated within the mitochondria and inhibit complex I activity, which leads to the decrease in ATP content and bring widespread damage to neurons. The inhibition of complex I is considered as the "primary injury" to dopaminergic neurons[38,39]. However, more attention have recently been drawn to the "secondary damage" to neurons caused by inflammatory processes which have been suggested to have a major impact on the progressive dopaminergic cell death in PD[38-40].

The hallmark of neuroinflammation in PD is the activation of microglia. From a neuropathological standpoint, microglial activation is indicative of an active, ongoing process of cell death[40,41]. Activated microglia not only bring damage to neurons through releasing a variety of noxious compounds[42,43], but also recruit and activate more microglial cells, forming a vicious cycle that leads to more dopaminergic neuronal death. In the present study, after $MPP^{+}$ intoxication to SN, we observed a progressive TH-positive cell loss and behavioral defects in rats, which were consistent with previous studies[23,31,44]. Activation of microglia was seen from the third day after $MPP^{+}$ injection and lasted throughout our experiment. Together with the suggestion that in the etiology of PD, activation of microglia represent an important cause of dopaminergic neuronal death[7,39], so it is postulated that microglia inhibitors might protect dopaminergic cell from injury induced by PD neurotoxins.

Extracts of the herb TWHF have been used for over two centuries as Traditional Chinese Medicine (TCM) to treat a variety of inflammatory and autoimmune diseases. Most of the pharmacological activity of TWHF can be attributed to triptolide and its most abundant and active component[14,45]. Here, we showed that chronic administration of triptolide decreased the immunodensity of OX-42, attenuated TH-positive neuronal loss and ameliorated the behavioral abnormalities in $MPP^{+}$-induced hemiparkinsonian rats. Our results are in agreement with previous reports, wherein triptolide inhibits LPS-induced microglial activation and dopaminergic neuronal loss[13,16,17], providing further evidence for the involvement of microglia in PD pathogenesis and the therapeutic potential for microglia inhibitors.

One of the possible mechanisms underlying the pharmaceutical effect of triptolide may be suppressing the expression of cyclooxygenase-2 (Cox-2), a specific proinflammatory factor which has emerged as an important mediator of microglial activation[40]. Neurons expressing COX-2 would cause their own demise through a harmful interplay with microglia[46-48]. Studies using COX-2 knockout mice and COX-2 inhibitors demonstrated reduced microglial activation and attenuated dopaminergic cell loss in PD models[40,49,50]. Since triptolide have been suggested to inhibit COX-2 expression in a variety of settings[14,51], further researches are warranted to determine whether triptolide exerts its inhibitory effect on microglial activation in $MPP^+$ rat model of PD through modulating COX-2 expression.

It is also worth mentioning that inhibition of microglia by triptolide, as used here, only partially blocked the dopaminergic cell death, suggesting that other mechanisms independent of microglia-related neuronal damage are also involved in $MPP^+$ neurotoxicity. As mentioned above, after $MPP^+$ is taken up by dopaminergic neurons, it is concentrated in mitochondria and inhibits complex I, resulting in ATP depletion and subsequent cell death[52]. Thus, the inhibition of complex I may account for another aspect of the disease phenotype which cannot be ameliorated by microglia inhibitors. Although this possibility cannot be confirmed with certainty, our observation that inhibition of microglia by triptolide preserve only a part of TH-positive neurons from injury rather support the view that dopaminergic neurons are damaged through more than one mechanism.

In summary, our result support the involvement of microglia in the progressive dopaminergic neuronal loss in $MPP^+$ rat model of PD. Triptolide exerted neuroprotective effect on $MPP^+$-induced dopaminergic neuronal injury and attenuated behavioral disabilities. Suppression of microglial activation may, at least in part, account for the mechanism underlying the neuroprotective effect of triptolide. Control of microglia-related neuroinflammation, thus, may represent a promising therapeutic strategy in the future management of PD.

*Acknowledgments*: This work was supported by National Great Project of Scientific and Technical Supporting Programs Funded by Ministry of Science and Technology of China during the 11th Five-year Plan (No. 2006BAI04A11-3), Foundation of Doctor Unit at High School from Ministry of Education (No. 20060246072), Medical Leader Sponsorship by Shanghai Municipal Government (No. 2007-057).

## References


[1] de Lau LML, Breteler MMB. Epidemiology of Parkinson's disease. Lancet Neurol 2006, 5: 525-535.

[2] Lang AE, Lozano AM. Parkinson's disease. First of two parts. N Engl J Med 1998, 339: 1044-1053.

[3] Zhang HL, Wu JJ, Ren HM, Wang J, Su YR, Jiang YP. Therapeutic effect of microencapsulated porcine retinal pigmented epithelial cells transplantation on rat model of Parkinson's disease. Neurosci Bull 2007, 23: 137-144.

[4] Poewe W. The need for neuroprotective therapies in Parkinson's disease. Neurology 2006, 66: S2-S9.

[5] Hauser RA, Zesiewicz TA. Clinical trials aimed at detecting neuroprotection in Parkinson's disease. Neurology 2006, 66: S58-S68.

[6] Ouchi Y, Yoshikawa E, Sekine Y, Futatsubashi M, Kanno T, Ogusu T, *et al.* Microglial activation and dopamine terminal loss in early Parkinson's disease. Ann Neurol 2005, 57: 168-175.

[7] Kim YS, Joh TH. Microglia, major player in the brain inflammation: their roles in the pathogenesis of Parkinson's disease. Exp Mol Med 2006, 38: 333-347.

[8] Whitton PS. Inflammation as a causative factor in the aetiology of Parkinson's disease. Br J Pharmacol 2007, 150: 963-976.

[9] Langston JW, Forno LS, Tetrud J, Reeves AG, Kaplan JA, Karluk D. Evidence of active nerve cell degeneration in the substantia nigra of humans years after 1-methyl-4-phenyl-1,2,3,6-tetrahydropyridine exposure. Ann Neurol 1999, 46: 598-605.

[10] McGeer PL, Schwab C, Parent A, Doudet D. Presence of reactive microglia in monkey substantia nigra years after 1-methyl-4-phenyl-1,2,3,6-tetrahydropyridine administration. Ann Neurol 2003, 54: 599-604.

[11] Cicchetti F, Brownell AL, Williams K, Chen YI, Livni E, Isacson O. Neuroinflammation of the nigrostriatal pathway during progressive 6-OHDA dopamine degeneration in rats monitored by immunohistochemistry and PET imaging. Eur J Neurosci 2002, 15: 991-998.

[12] Yuan H, Zheng JC, Liu P, Zhang SF, Xu JY, Bai LM. Pathogenesis of Parkinson's disease: oxidative stress, environmental impact factors and inflammatory processes. Neurosci Bull 2007, 23: 125-130.

[13] Qiu D, Kao PN. Immunosuppressive and anti-inflammatory mechanisms of triptolide, the principal active diterpenoid from the Chinese medicinal herb Tripterygium wilfordii Hook. f. Drugs R D 2003, 4: 1-18.

[14] Ma J, Dey M, Yang H, Poulev A, Pouleva R, Dorn R, *et al.* Anti-inflammatory and immunosuppressive compounds from Tripterygium wilfordii. Phytochemistry 2007, 68: 1172-1178.

[15] Liu QY, Chen TY, Chen GY, Shu XL, Sun A, Ma PC, *et al.* Triptolide impairs dendritic cell migration by inhibiting CCR7 and COX-2 expression through PI3-K/Akt and NF-kappa B pathways. Mol Immunol 2007, 44: 2686-2696.

[16] Li FQ, Lu XZ, Liang XB, Zhou HF, Xue B, Liu XY, *et al.* Triptolide, a Chinese herbal extract, protects dopaminergic neurons from inflammation-mediated damage through inhibition of microglial activation. J Neuroimmunol 2004, 148: 24-31.

[17] Zhou HF, Liu XY, Niu DB, Li FQ, He QH, Wang XM. Triptolide protects dopaminergic neurons from inflammation-mediated damage lipopolysaccharide intranigral induced by injection. Neurobiol Dis 2005, 18: 441-449.

[18] Maharaj DS, Saravanan KS, Maharaj H, Mohanakumar KP, Daya S. Acetaminophen and aspirin inhibit superoxide anion generation and lipid peroxidation, and protect against 1-methyl-4-phenyl pyridinium-induced dopaminergic neurotoxicity in rats. Neurochem Int 2004, 44: 355-360.

[19] Paxinos G, Watson C. The rat brain in stereotaxic coordinates. 5th ed. 2005, Sydney: Elsevier Academic Press.

[20] Truong L, Allbutt H, Kassiou M, Henderson JM. Developing a preclinical model of Parkinson's disease: a study of behaviour in rats with graded 6-OHDA lesions. Behav Brain Res 2006, 169: 1-9.

[21] Olsson M, Nikkhah G, Bentlage C, Bjorklund A. Forelimb akinesia in the rat Parkinson model: differential effects of dopamine agonists and nigral transplants as assessed by a new stepping test. J Neurosci 1995, 15: 3863-3875.

[22] Tillerson JL, Cohen AD, Philhower J, Miller GW, Zigmond MJ, Schallert T. Forced limb-use effects on the behavioral and neurochemical effects of 6-hydroxydopamine. J Neurosci 2001, 21: 4427-4435.

[23] Tillerson JL, Caudle WM, Reveron ME, Miller GW. Exercise induces behavioral recovery and attenuates neurochemical deficits in rodent models of Parkinson's disease. Neuroscience 2003, 119: 899-911.

[24] Hua Y, Schallert T, Keep RF, Wu JM, Hoff JT, Xi GH. Behavioral tests after intracerebral hemorrhage in the rat. Stroke 2002, 33: 2478-2484.

[25] Monville C, Torres EM, Dunnett SB. Validation of the l-dopa-induced dyskinesia in the 6-OHDA model and evaluation of the effects of selective dopamine receptor agonists and antagonists. Brain Res Bull 2005, 68: 16-23.

[26] Sun S, Cao H, Han M, Li TT, Pan HL, Zhao ZQ, *et al.* New evidence for the involvement of spinal fractalkine receptor in pain facilitation and spinal glial activation in rat model of monoarthritis. Pain 2007, 129: 64-75.

[27] Vaananen AJ, Rauhala P, Tuominen RK, Liesi P. KDI tripeptide of gamma 1 laminin protects rat dopaminergic neurons from 6-OHDA induced toxicity. J Neurosci Res 2006, 84: 655-665.

[28] Liu B, Hong JS. Role of microglia in inflammation-mediated neurodegenerative diseases: Mechanisms and strategies for therapeutic intervention. J Pharmacol Exp Ther 2003, 304: 1-7.

[29] Miwa H, Kubo T, Morita S, Nakanishi I, Kondo T. Oxidative stress and microglial activation in substantia nigra following striatal $MPP^+$. Neuroreport 2004, 15: 1039-1044.

[30] Deumens R, Blokland A, Prickaerts J. Modeling Parkinson's disease in rats: an evaluation of 6-OHDA lesions of the nigrostriatal pathway. Exp Neurol 2002, 175: 303-317.

[31] Banerjee R, Sreetama S, Saravanan KS, Dey SN, Mohanakumar KP. Apoptotic mode of cell death in substantia nigra following intranigral infusion of the parkinsonian neurotoxin, $MPP^+$ in sprague-dawley rats: Cellular, molecular and ultrastructural evidences. Neurochem Res 2007, 32: 1238-1247.

[32] Du YS, Ma ZZ, Lin SZ, Dodel RC, Gao F, Bales KR, et al. Minocycline prevents nigrostriatal dopaminergic neurodegeneration in the MPTP model of Parkinson's disease. Proc Natl Acad Sci U S A 2001, 98: 14669-14674.

[33] Wu DC, Jackson-Lewis V, Vila M, Tieu K, Teismann P, Vadseth C, *et al.* Blockade of microglial activation is neuroprotective in the 1-methyl-4-phenyl-1,2,3,6-tetrahydropyridine mouse model of Parkinson disease. J Neurosci 2002, 22: 1763-1771.

[34] Langston JW, Ballard P, Tetrud JW, Irwin I. Chronic Parkinsonism in humans due to a product of meperidine-analog synthesis. Science 1983, 219: 979-980.

[35] Chen XW, Sun SG, Cheng DB, Tian YY. Overexpression of 14-3-3 protein protects pheochromocytoma cells against 1-methyl-4-phenylpyridinium toxicity. Neurosci Bull 2006, 22: 281-287.

[36] Samantaray S, Chandra G, Mohanakumar KP. Calcium channel agonist, (+/-)-Bay K8644, causes a transient increase in striatal monoamine oxidase activity in Balb/c mice. Neurosci Lett 2003, 342: 73-76.

[37] Przedborski S, Vila M. The 1-methyl-4-phenyl-1,2,3,6-tetrahydropyridine mouse model: a tool to explore the pathogenesis of Parkinson's disease. Ann N Y Acad Sci 2003, 991: 189-198.

[38] Hunot S, Hirsch EC. Neuroinflammatory processes in Parkinson's disease. Ann Neurol 2003, 53: S49-S58.

[39] Hirsch EC, Hunot S, Hartmann A. Neuroinflammatory processes in Parkinson's disease. Parkinsonism Relat Disord 2005, 11: S9-S15.

[40] Vijitruth R, Liu M, Choi DY, Nguyen XV, Hunter RL, Bing G. Cyclooxygenase-2 mediates microglial activation and secondary dopaminergic cell death in the mouse MPTP model of Parkinson's disease. J Neuroinflammation, 2006, 3: 6.

[41] Kim SU, de Vellis J. Microglia in health and disease. J Neurosci Res 2005, 81: 302-313.

[42] Teismann P, Tieu K, Cohen O, Choi DK, Wu DC, Marks D, *et al.* Pathogenic role of glial cells in Parkinson's disease. Mov Disord 2003, 18: 121-129.

[43] Youdim MB, Grunblatt E, Levites Y, Maor G, Mandel S. Early and late molecular events in neurodegeneration and neuroprotection in Parkinson's disease MPTP model as assessed by cDNA microarray; the role of iron. Neurotox Res 2002, 4: 679-689.

[44] Goralski KB, Renton KW. Brain inflammation enhances 1-methyl-4-phenylpyridinium-evoked neurotoxicity in rats. Toxicol Appl Pharmacol 2004, 196: 381-389.

[45] Zhu XZ, Li XY, Liu J. Recent pharmacological studies on natural products in China. Eur J Pharmacol 2004, 500: 221-230.

[46] Teismann P, Tieu K, Choi DK, Wu DC, Naini A, Hunot S, *et al.* Cyclooxygenase-2 is instrumental in Parkinson's disease neurodegeneration. Proc Natl Acad Sci U S A 2003, 100: 5473-5478.

[47] Wang TG, Pei Z, Zhang W, Liu B, Langenbach R, Lee C, *et al.* $MPP^+$-induced COX-2 activation and subsequent dopaminergic neurodegeneration. FASEB J 2005, 19: 1134-1136.

[48] Shie FS, Montine KS, Breyer RM, Montine TJ. Microglial EP2 is critical to neurotoxicity from activated cerebral innate immunity. Glia 2005, 52: 70-77.

[49] Feng ZH, Wang TG, Li DD, Fung P, Wilson BC, Liu B, *et al.* Cyclooxygenase-2-deficient mice are resistant to 1-methyl-4-phenyl1,2,3,6-tetrahydropyridine-induced damage of dopaminergic neurons in the substantia nigra. Neurosci Lett 2002, 329: 354-358.

[50] Sanchez-Pernaute R, Ferree A, Cooper O, Yu M, Brownell AL, Isacson O. Selective COX-2 inhibition prevents progressive dopamine neuron degeneration in a rat model of Parkinson's disease. J Neuroinflammation 2004, 1: 6.
[51] Dai YQ, Jin DZ, Zhu XZ, Lei DL. Triptolide inhibits COX-2 expression via NF-kappa B pathway in astrocytes. Neurosci Res 2006, 55: 154-160.
[52] Schober A. Classic toxin-induced animal models of Parkinson's disease: 6-OHDA and MPTP. Cell Tissue Res 2004, 318: 215-224.

Andrea Riegel

# Heart and Kidney – li ☲ and kan ☵ An Extraordinary Yin-Yang Couple in Chinese Philosophy and Medicine

## Introduction

In Chinese medicine the heart and kidney have an extraordinary relationship. The heart is the ruler organ while the kidney in its role as a minister serves and controls the heart. In the cycle of the Five Phases the heart represents the phase of fire whereas the kidney represents the phase of water and water controls fire, as we know. But this is not all about the relationships between heart and kidney. What makes the relationship between heart and kidney so extraordinary? Are these ideas concerning the relationship between heart and kidney mere nonsense or is there even any logic to them that we can make use of?

When we look closer at the theories not only concerning kidney and heart but concerning Chinese medicine in general we find out that most theories concerning the system of inner organs and their correlations have their origin in the Book of Changes.

## 1. The Book of Changes (Yijing)

The Book of Changes is the source book for all Chinese sciences including medicine. So we must take a look at this work. The basic canon is composed of 64 hexagrams with little commentaries. These 64 hexagrams have their basis in eight different trigrams forming four Yin-yang couples. They are composed of the symbols for sun ⚊ and moon ⚋, light and shadow. The basic idea was to draw a picture of heaven and earth and to trace the path of sun and moon during a year by means of line symbols. It was written during the Yin-Shang Dynasty (1401-1137 B.C.). During the Spring and Autumn (790-476 B.C.) periods and the Warring States (475-221 B.C.) ten different commentaries on this book came into existence dealing with different aspects of the hexagrams and the basic trigrams. Some of them are influenced by Confucian ethics – and for this reason – give a moral interpretation of the text. The commentaries that mostly influenced Chinese medicine are the Great Appendix (*xici-zhuan*) and the *shuogua* commentary which described the trigrams, their qualities and the relationships between the trigrams.

There are three basic ideas that can be identified in the commentaries and which deeply influenced Chinese medical theories:

1. There exists an endless cycle of production and reproduction, heaven and earth being father and mother of all things and man´s main duty on earth is to try to imitate the virtue of heaven and earth.
2. Heaven, earth and man are the three potentials (*sancai* 三才), man is a copy of heaven and earth and therefore a microcosm in macrocosm.
3. The world is divided into two opposite poles Yin and Yang.[1]

As for production and reproduction we find in the Great Appendix a world creation theory very similar to that we find in the book of *Laozi.* It reads: "(…) the original One *Taiji* makes the two basic forms, these two basic forms make the four symbols (*sixiang* 四象), the four symbols make the eight trigrams "[2].

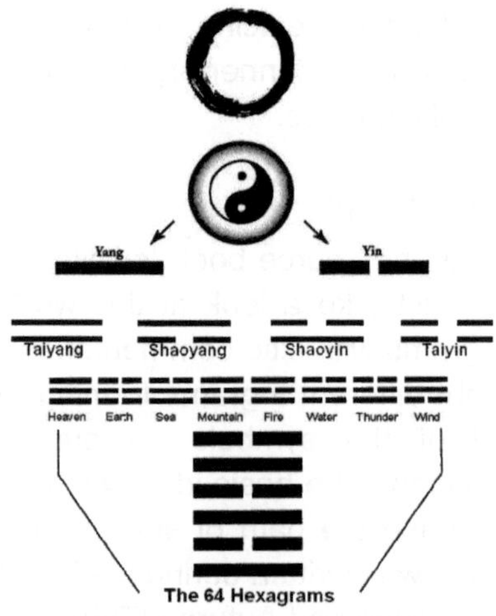


Illustration 1 the Yijing world creation theory

1 This idea is firmly rooted in the *shuogua* commentary.

2 Zhouyi zhezhong (2003): 894

We also find the description of two different arrangements of the trigrams as a cycle: the map of the "former heaven" known as Hetu 河图(map of the He river) that represents the universe before the material world came into existence and the map of the "later heaven" known as Luoshu 洛书 (scripture of the Luo river) that represents the world. We will discuss them in the next chapter.

## 1.1 The Trigrams

The above mentioned arrangements of Hetu and Luoshu represent the universe before and after the existence of the material world. In the Hetu the so called map of the "former heaven" the opposite trigrams occupy opposite positions. Starting from the highest Yin (*kun*) ☷ and turning to the left which is the way of Yang we see Yang ascending towards the extreme Yang (*qian*) ☰ and then falling direction beginning Yin and culminating in the utmost Yin which is *kun*. The symbols of rising sun and rising moon are very clear in this map.

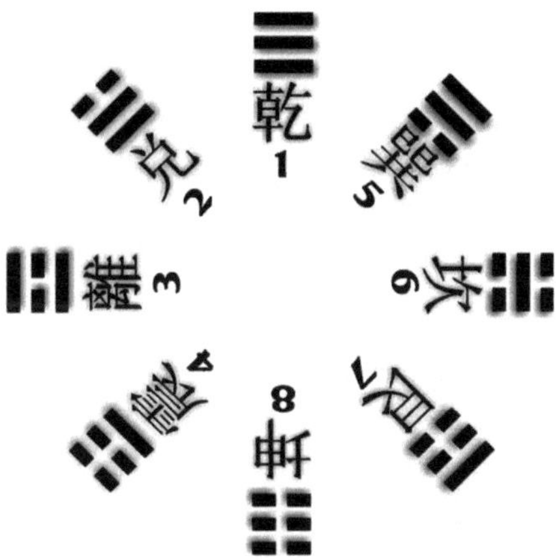


Illustration 2 The Hetu map

For the formation of the material world represented in the map of the later heaven there must be a movement in every trigram. The ideas concerning these movements are complicated and vary in the *Yijing* reception. We do not need to talk about the movements in detail, we can consider the map as a whole.[1] The most interesting feature in this map is that in the pole positions north and south we find the trigrams *kan* and *li*, the only two opposite trigrams in this map occupying opposite positions.

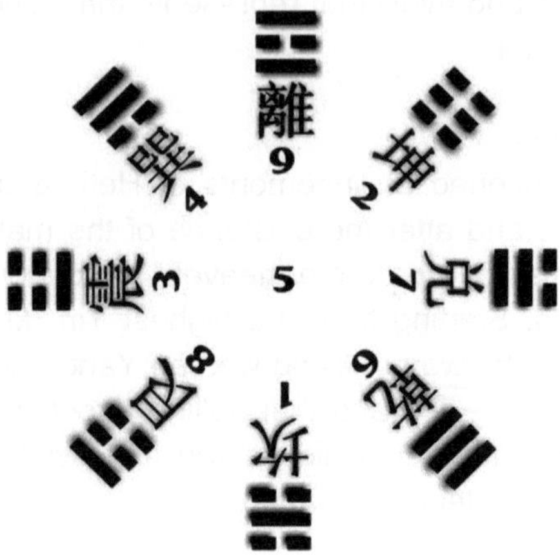


Illustration 2: The Luoshu map

As the earth is supposed to be a copy of heaven it is also logical that the trigrams not only represent constellations of sun and moon but also symbolize manifestations in the material world and their corresponding characteristics. The *shuogua* commentary describes the following correspondences:

| | | |
|---|---|---|
| Heaven | ☰ qian | Strength |
| Earth | ☷ kun | Devotion receptiveness |
| Thunder | ☳ zhen | Movement |
| Wind | ☴ sun | Soft Penetration |
| Water | ☵ kan | Falling, Danger |
| Fire | ☲ li | Brilliance |
| Mountain | ☶ gen | Stability |
| Sea | ☱ dui | Joy |

1 For further details see H. Bohn (1998).

Because the Book of Changes identifies heaven, earth and man as one entity the *shuogua* commentary describes the correspondences of trigrams with structures of the human body and inner organs. For example:

| Qian ☰ Heaven | Kun ☷ Earth | Zhen ☳ Thunder | Sun ☴ Wind | Kan ☵ Water | Li ☲ Fire | Gen ☶ Moun-tain | Dui ☱ Sea |
|---|---|---|---|---|---|---|---|
| Lung | Stomach | Gallbladder | Liver | Kidney | Heart | Spleen | Small Intestine |
| Head | Abdomen | Foot | Thigh | Ear Blood | Eyes | Hand | Mouth |

As earth and mountain are identical in their material substance and as a sea consists of water the eight trigrams and their correspondences may be summed up in the Five Phases:

| | | | | |
|---|---|---|---|---|
| *Li*<br>Fire | *Kan*<br>Water<br>*Dui*<br>Sea | *Zhen*<br>Thunder<br>*Sun*<br>Wind | *Kun*<br>Earth<br>*Gen*<br>Mountain | *Qian*<br>Heaven |
| Fire | Water | Wood | Earth | Metal |
| Heart | Kidney<br>Small int. | Gallbladder<br>Liver | Spleen<br>Stomach | Lung |

We find correspondences which are, in part, very similar to those we find in Chinese medicine. Let us focus on the two trigrams *kan* and *li*.

### 1.1.1 Kan 坎 ☵ and Li 离 ☲

*Kan* and *li* are opposite trigrams. *Kan* has one Yang line between two Yin lines, *li* has one Yin line between two Yang lines. The correspondences we find in the Book of Changes, that is in the *shuogua* commentary, as follows:

- *Kan*: Water, kidney, ear, blood
- *Li*: fire, heart, eyes

There are even more correspondences for *kan* and the kidneys hidden in the Book of Changes. *Kan* is located in the north, the north represents the winter. The *shuogua* commentary says: "*Kan* means water. It is the trigram exactly in the north, it is the trigram of trouble, all things have their origin in it."[1] From this commentary one may draw the conclusion that *kan*-kidney stands for the beginning and the end of life, birth and death. Even the main task of the kidney, the storage (*feng* 封)is included in this sentence because winter is the time of storage. Moreover the trouble mentioned in the commentary is an allusion to the fact that the kidney is responsible for the energy of all the other organs or, in other words, the other inner organs depend on the kidney´s energy.

The opposite trigram is *li* which means "brilliance". In the Luoshu map it is located in the south. This indicates that the corresponding inner organ has a tendency towards burning. The brilliance of the eyes reflects the state of consciousness, the consciousness *shen* represents the mental aspect of the heart. (see below 2.2). The trigram *li* symbolizes the sun and a lightning. In its brilliance *li* equals *qian*, whose place it takes over in the Luoshu. As it is hard outside and soft inside it can be compared to an oyster or to crustaceans in general. In the flora it symbolizes the empty stem of a tree. By its character the trigram *li* is highly Yang, nevertheless *li* represents a Yin-trigram whereas *kan* represents a Yang trigram.[2]

The intimate relationship between *li* and *kan* is also shown in the *shuogua* commentary as it states: "*Kan* is water, it is a linking channel, it is hidden, curved, its movement is straight-lined, in man trouble brings about danger, it means heart disease, ear pain, it is the blood trigram, it is purple red. In the horse it represents the marvelous back, palpitations of the heart, the head bent down, a weak leg, slow movement, as a carriage it

1 *Zhouyi zhezhong* (2003): 1012

2 The categorization is based on the fact that the trigram *li* is composed of two Yang lines and the number of "two" is not adequate for Yang.

has many defects, it is a ditch, it represents the moon and a fleeing robber. In a tree it is the stable heart."[1]

The responsibility for blood may be clear because the blood in the human body corresponds to the water on earth. We see trouble and tiredness on the one hand, stability on the other hand, represented in the stable heart of a tree and the strong back of a horse. Here the correspondence of the kidney with physical and mental stability is indicated. The character of *kan* is stable but very feeble at the same time. The direct relationship to the heart is illustrated because the *kan*-trigram stands for palpitation of the heart and heart disease (*xin bing* 心病). The pathology of the kidney must therefore be: heart disease and may be coronary heart disease caused by blood stasis, physical and mental exhaustion, sterility.

## 2. Kidney and Heart in Classical Medical Literature

The physical, physiological as well as the pathological aspects of kidneys and heart are already described in both parts of the *Huangdi neijing, Suwen* and *Lingshu*, and in the Classic of Difficult Issues, the *Nanjing*. The *Nanjing* focuses on the anatomy of the organs whereas the *Huangdi neijing* describes the correspondences in regard to the Five Phases' theory and aspects of the correlation between the organs.

### 2.1 The Kidney

In Chinese medicine the kidney is the most important inner organ. Its fundamental responsibility for the whole life process of man may be seen in the Chinese character for kidney "*shen*" 肾. In the lower part of the character we have the radical *rou* 肉 for "flesh". In the upper part there is *chen* 臣 for "minister" and you 又 for the right hand. This means that the kidney is a highly respected organ with direct contact to the ruler organ. It works as a servant and its function is as important as the work of a state´s minister. As he is the master of other ministers, the kidney needs other subordinate organs to fulfill its task. So the kidney is directly subordinate to the ruler: the heart. It is a solid base in the organism but needs the support of other organs.

*Suwen*, chap. (5) enumerates all correspondences of the kidney in the environment and human body, the most important in our context being

1 *Zhouyi zhezhong* (2003): 1024

the following: Water, cold, salty taste, black color, bones and marrow, blood, ears, fear, i.e. will. As we have seen these correspondences came into existence not only through mere convention, some of them can be derived directly from the Book of Changes.[1]

The kidney is responsible for the stability of the bones and nourishes the marrow, which also refers to the brain. So the intellectual power in part depends on the power of the kidneys. The *Lingshu* chap. (17) establishes the correspondence between the kidneys and the ears and states that the kidney-meridian passes through the ear. This is in fact a false statement. Either one wanted to confirm the statements of the Book of Changes or one had experiences which brought one to the conclusion that there must be a correlation between kidney and ear. As for the mental aspect one finds "the will" (*zhi* 志) lodging in a stable kidney or "the fear" (*kong* 恐) in a weak kidney.

As for the black color we see a difference to the Book of Changes. There the kidney´s color is purple red (*chi* 赤) because the blood has red color, the heart being "dark purple " (*dachi* 大赤). The color *hei* 黑 for "black" symbolizes directly the kidney´s function: Though *hei* is itself a radical (No. 203) it shows the fire below and "soot" above. So we can deduce the kidney´s function of warming of the organs and vaporization *Qihua* 氣化 because the kidney´s Qi ascends like vapor. If the kidney´s Qi is insufficient there will be no dampness for the body and consequently the blood and body fluids will dry up. Bloodstasis will be the result and stagnating blood is black.

Nonetheless the most important responsibility of the kidney – in our context – has to do with the sexual power and the reproduction of man. The basis for this correspondence may be, first of all, the fact that man normally has one of each of his vital organs but he has two kidneys, these two being a Yin-Yang pair.

---

1 There are still other philosophical works and their commentaries which may have played an important role in the correspondences. We may mention in this respect the Book of Rites (*Liji*), the chapter of the monthly calendar (*Yueling*) or the Great Plan (*Hongfan*) which is part of the *Shangshu*.

### 2.1.1 The "Gate of Life" mingmen 命門

The most amazing fact for the doctors in ancient times was that the kidney can be found twice in the body both the left and right side of the spine. So the 36th Difficult issue of the Classic of Difficult Issues (*Nanjing*) states: "(1) Each of the depots is a single [entity], except for the kidneys which represent a twin [entity]. Why is that so? (2) It is like this. The two kidneys are not both kidneys. The one on the left is the kidney; the one on the right is the gate of life. (3) The gate of life is the place where the spirit-essence lodges; it is the place to which the original influences are tied. (4) Hence, in males it stores the essence; in females it holds the womb. (5) Hence, one knows that there is only one kidney."[1] These lines tell us that the kidneys are a pair, a Yin-Yang couple which can produce new life. In this text the left side kidney represents the Yang aspect whereas the right side kidney represents Yin because it stores our sexual essence.[2] The *mingmen* is the material base for the fulfillment of the "decree of heaven" that is the duty to produce descendants.

In the Ming Dynasty's "Illustrated and Commented Classic of Difficult Issues" (*Tuzhu Nanjing*) by Zhang Shixian we find an illustration of the *mingmen*. We see Hexagram 64 ("before the completion") on top and Hexagram (63) ("the completion") below, the two opposite Hexagrams where *li* and *kan* are united (see illustration 4, next page).[3]

This means that fire and water brought together create new life. The original idea is that in the Luoshu *kan* and *li* are mother and father of all things of the world and these trigrams take over the area of heaven *qian* and earth *kun* in the map of the former heaven Hetu.

1 Unschuld (1986): 382

2 The categorization of Yin and Yang changed during Chinese medical history. In the Ming dynasty (1360-1644) an important discussion came up about the meaning and the location of the *mingmen*.

3 *Tuzhu Nanjing* (1991): 124

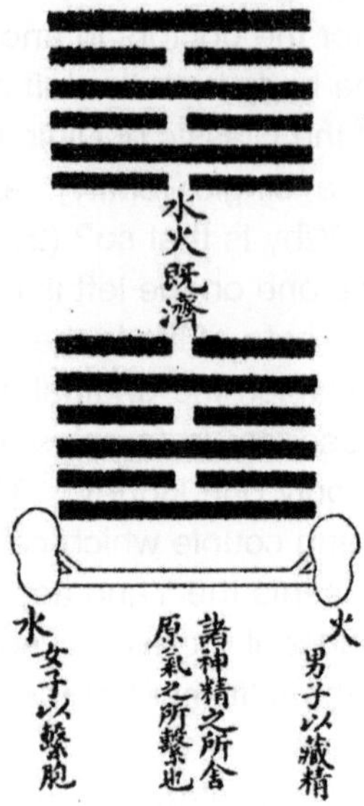
水火既濟
火
男子以藏精
諸神精之所舍
原氣之所繫也
水
女子以繫胞

Illustration 4 The mingmen in the Tuzhu Nanjing

2.2 The heart

The heart is represented by a very simple character *xin* 心 that shows the shape of the heart and three blood drops. It is the ruler organ in the organism and located in the upper burner that is in the Yang district of the body. Although it is a Yin-organ like the kidney regarding its character the heart is Yang.

As for all depots *Suwen*, chap. (5)[1] enumerates all correspondences of the heart in environment and human body, the most important in our context being the following: Fire, heat, bitter taste, red color, blood vessels, blood, spirit (*shen* 神), joy (xi 喜).

*Suwen* chap. (5) stresses the heart's responsibility for blood. It says that the heart "brings about" the blood (*sheng xue* 生血) meaning that the red color of blood is bestowed by the heart. And the heart is responsible for the blood vessels. This ultimately means that the power of heart-Qi is responsible for the blood circulation all over the body. The heart is ex-

1 See *Suwen* (5); Yang Weijie (1990): 50

tremely sensible to stimuli and very easily weakened by (sexual) desires. If the *shen*-aspect, the aspect of consciousness, is harmed for example by excess of desires then severe mental disturbances will be the consequences. For this reason it is like this the heart absolutely needs control by another organ that is the kidney.

## 2.3 Physiological and Pathological Relationships between Heart and Kidney

In the cycle of the Five Phases the relation between heart and kidney as representatives of fire and water is that of control meaning that water has to control fire. We also know that there is not only the control exerted by water but that there is a real mutual interaction, a correlation, between the two organs which in classical literature reads "heart and kidney are in communication with one another" (*xin shen xiang jiao* 心肾相交) or, as *Suwen* chap. (81) states "water and fire touch one another (shui huo xiang gan 水火相感). One can also read "water and fire nourish each other" (*shui huo xiang ji* 水火相济). One may understand the correlations of *jiao* 交 and *ji* 济 as being on a physical level whereas the word "*gan*" 感 "touch" which writes with the radical for "heart" *xin* 心 shows that there is even an emotional aspect in the correlation between heart and kidney, heart and kidney come into contact by virtue of their mental aspects *shen* (heart), "spirit", and *zhi* (kidney), "will". As the character for *zhi* 志 already shows the heart is closely correlated to the mental aspect of the kidney because in the lower part we have the radical for "heart", *xin* 心.

### 2.3.1 Physiological Relationships

The first relationship between heart and kidney is established by the meridians: kidney and heart meridians are both shaoyin-meridians, the kidney-meridian being called foot-shaoyin and the heart-meridian representing hand-shaoyin. In practice one may use this fact to reestablish the contact between heart and kidney.

As we have seen the kidney is a minister serving the ruler organ the heart. At same time it has to control the ruler, a point of view which corresponds to the Five Phases´ cycle of control. Moreover as in a state´s government the relationship between ruler and minister is a mutual one: the ruler himself takes care of his ministers. The same rule is valid for the organs: heart-yang descends in order to warm kidney-Yang while on the other hand kidney-water meaning all aspects of the kidney-function (Yin, Yang and Qi) ascend to nourish heart-Yin or to control heart-Yang. That is what is meant by "heart and kidney are in communication with one another" or "water and fire nourish one another". Even the aspect of "touch" on a physical level is included here.

Furthermore both organs, heart and kidney, have a connection to blood. The kidney governs the blood production whereas the heart governs the blood circulation. Kidney and heart govern the outer part of the body (*wai* 外) and the inner (*nei* 内) respectively, meaning, as stated in *Suwen*, chap. (52)[1], that the kidney is responsible for the inner – mental – stability whereas the heart by means of its *shen*-aspect establishes the contact between man and his environment.[2] On the other hand the *shen*-aspect of the heart can only be stable as long as heart-blood is sufficient and sufficiency of heart-blood ultimately depends on the kidney. We may therefore imagine and summarize the relationships between heart and kidney as a single Yin-Yang symbol:

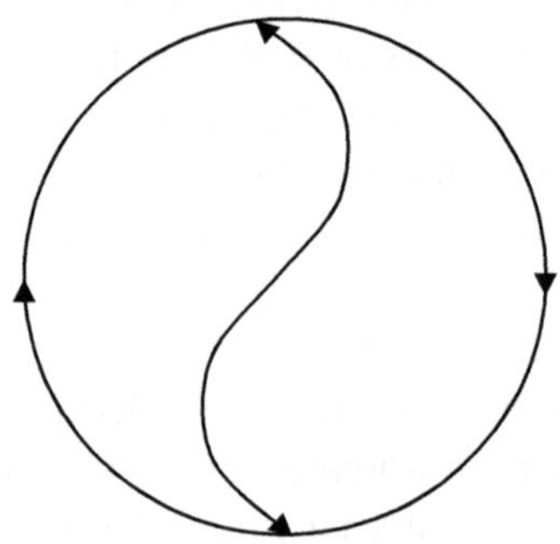


The "Introduction to medicine" (*Yixue rumen*) of the Ming Dynasty divides the heart into two parts: one physical and one spiritual mental. It states:

1 See *Suwen* (52); Yang Weijie (1990): 380

2 The *Lingshu* chap. (36) however defines the outer part of the body as correspondence to the kidney. See *Lingshu yishi* (1997): 248. In this sense it means that the kidney is responsible for the hardness of the bones.

"The heart is the ruler in the body, there is a heart consisting of flesh and blood looking like the bud of a lotus flower located beneath the lung and above the liver; and there is the spiritual heart, spirit is what Qi and blood change, the root of life (...) it has no material existence, it governs all things, it has no substance, it is spiritual and tasteless; but physical and spiritual heart are one entity."[1] Here one can see that the kidney is the physical root of life while the heart is the spiritual root of life.

2.3.2 Pathological Relationships between Heart and Kidney

Disturbances of the harmony between heart and kidney are those where "heart and kidney are not in communication with one another" or where "kidney water does not control heart fire". Hyperactivity of heart-fire or weakness of kidney-water will result in a disruption of the communication between the two organs and this will produce physical and mental effects. The clinical symptoms are in most cases those of "blazing heart-fire" or insufficiency of heart-Yin. In severe cases there may be serious mental and physical symptoms like neurosis, mania, hysteria, fear and nightmares, or simply insomnia or nervousness, palpitations, high diastolic or systolic blood pressure, headache, dizziness, flushed face, hard pulse, eye pain, symptoms that are possibly related to high tension of sympathetic nerves. In western medicine we know very well that high blood pressure may harm the glomeruli in the kidneys and that, on the other hand, nephropathy may result in high blood pressure.

The *Yixue rumen* goes so far to say that original heart diseases *xinbing* 心病 do not exist. It must be that either disease of the kidneys was transmitted to the heart or mental disturbances such as fear or melancholy opened the heart to pathogens.[2] This statement stresses the correlation between heart and kidney and the important role of the kidney for the heart´s health.

3. Conclusion

As we have seen many aspects of the inner organs that are still valid in traditional Chinese medicine are described in the Book of Changes and therefore have their origin in philosophical ideas. From the point of view of

---

1 *Yixue rumen* (1995): 59

2 *Yixue rumen* (1995): 59

western medicine, we may accept various aspects of the inner organs as seen in Chinese medicine. We have observed the heart and kidney and we must confess that the ideas of Chinese medicine concerning the responsibilities of these two organs and the relationship between them are not mere nonsense. Through western medicine we can understand that the kidney is the basic organ for the production of new blood cells through the secretion of erythropoetine, we know that the kidneys are involved in calcium metabolism which is a very important base for the hardness of bones. We know that many nephrotoxic drugs are at the same time ototoxic and we also know that a low clearance rate of the kidneys may have negative effects on the brain, that high blood pressure may harm the glomeruli, and, that on the other hand nephropathy may be responsible for high blood pressure.

We may ask ourselves why philosophical ideas can be a basis for medical ideas or even treatments. The reason may be that consciousness plays an important part in the art of healing in several ethno-medical systems. The healers are aware of the fact that they do treat human beings and individuals, not only diseases and that the medical doctor is a medium who can make use not only of remedies but also of his own consciousness. Western medicine only focuses on standards and the so called "evidence based" medicine but in many cases consciousness may be the key to success.

When we return to our example and the practices in Chinese medicine, we can state that prevention plays an important role in Chinese medicine. So the recommendation for preventing heart disease and high blood pressure is to nourish both organs heart and kidney the crucial factors being life style and nutrition. Asceticism and "little desire" (*guayu* 寡欲) is the way to calm the heart and to nourish kidney-essence. As for nutrition we should prefer food which is neither too "hot" nor too "cold" in temperature, drink warm water and eat warm meals for the kidneys, protect the kidneys against cold and windy weather. These recommendations completely differ from Western medicine's way.

Generally speaking it may be not a mistake to combine the Chinese medicine´s point of view with the knowledge of Western medicine: that is, one should take into consideration the organism as one entity in which there are correlations between the inner organs, bearing in mind the fact that every human being is an individual and shows individual reactions, finding out the origin of a disease or a symptom and to begin treatment at the origin of the disease instead of merely treating symptoms. We should also take into consideration the fact that psychology and consciousness are an important factor in the healing process. The knowledge contained in western medicine and the conscious use of any natural healing art may make combined ethno and western medicine the perfect healing art.

## References


Bohn, Hermann G. (1998). Die Rezeption des Zhouyi in der chinesischen Philosophie, von den Anfängen bis zur Song-Dynastie. München: Herbert Utz.

Huang Shouqi. Zhouyi yizhu (Translated and commented edition of the Zhouyi) (1989). Shanghai: Gujian chubanshe.

*Lingshu yishi* (Translated and interpreted edition of the *Lingshu* (1997). Shanghai: Kexue jishu chubanshe.

Riegel, Andrea (2004). Diabetes und TCM. Munich: Pflaum.

Riegel, Andrea (2008). Die Niere shen. Klassische Konzepte der chinesischen Medizin im Lichte der modernen Schulmedizin. (Unpublished doctoral dissertation).

Riegel, Andrea (2008). Ling Zhen. Der geistig-spirituelle Weg der Akupunktur. Hochheim: Comed.

Ross, Jeremy (1995). Zang Fu. The System of Inner Organs in Chinese Medicine Uelzen: Medizinisch Literarische Gesellschaft.

Unschuld, Paul (1986). Nan-Ching. The Classic of Difficult Issues. Taipei: Southern Materials Center.

Wilder, G.D., J.H. Ingrim (1922). Analysis of Chinese Characters. Taipei: Caves Books LTD.

Yang Weijie (1990): Huangdi neijing Suwen yijie (Translsated and commented edition of the Simple Questions of the Yellow Emperor´s Classic of internal medicine). Taipei.

Yixue rumen (Introduction to medicine) (1995). Beijing: Zhongguo zhongyiyao chuban she.

Zhang Jiebin (2000). Leijing (The Yellow Emperor´s Classic of internal medicine in categories). Beijing: Zhongguo zhongyiya chuban she.

*Zhouyi zhezhong* (Analyse des Yijing) (2002). Beijing: Jiuzhou chubanshe.

Hua Zou

# The Time of Integrative Medicine

Classical Chinese Medicine regards a human being as a holistic being. In diagnosis and therapy the human being is thus positioned in a geographic, temporary, environmental and cultural field. School medicine and CCM have many methods in common, but CCM differs from classical medicine when it comes to pre-diagnosis which is based on the specific situation of the individual while following the principles of nature. Diseases appear at specific times, under special living conditions, at a certain age, and in certain climatic regions. Our body permanently changes its cell structure on a daily basis; all physical regulations have their own rhythm of time. Time is the essential factor of our lives and I will refer to some aspects that illustrate in which way CCM diagnosis and therapy are dependent on the factor of time.

## 1. An example of acupuncture treatment

At Christmas I met a young lady. She had weight problems, was pale, in a bad mood and suffered from constant headaches. I gave her my business card and asked her to visit me. And indeed, she came to my medical practice. After a comprehensive CCM diagnosis I started with the treatment. The headache disappeared immediately thereafter. Basically, I could have ended the therapy. But since CCM is a holistic therapy and seeks to eliminate the root cause of the symptoms I continued therapy. Especially, since the young woman also suffered from tiredness, back pain and menstruation problems. Another problem had been her gaining weight. I treated her only with acupuncture and cupping, without tablets or herbal tea, and her health improved soon after.

Nevertheless I noticed that my therapy was not ideal and that the lady still suffered from mental problems. She was very irritable and constantly angry. So I invited her to visit my health seminar. After my lessons in CCM she understood the underlying reasons for her problems and that these reasons had been presenting an obstacle to the therapeutic effect. The patient corrected her behaviour in her daily life and all of a sudden her medical symptoms improved. I employed my CCM regulation therapy in specific intervals, i.e. we took breaks after each therapy phase. After some time had passed, I repeated the tongue and pulse diagnosis and then adapted my treatment to the diagnosis, as I always do.

One year later the result was perfect: The lady was free from disorders, full of energy and her power of concentration had improved considerably. Her attainment in school was excellent, her mathematics grade was now 1.5 (A-) compared to 4 (D) a year ago where she had failed the test. Her average mark was a good 2.2. She reduced her weight, is mentally well balanced and full of self-confidence.

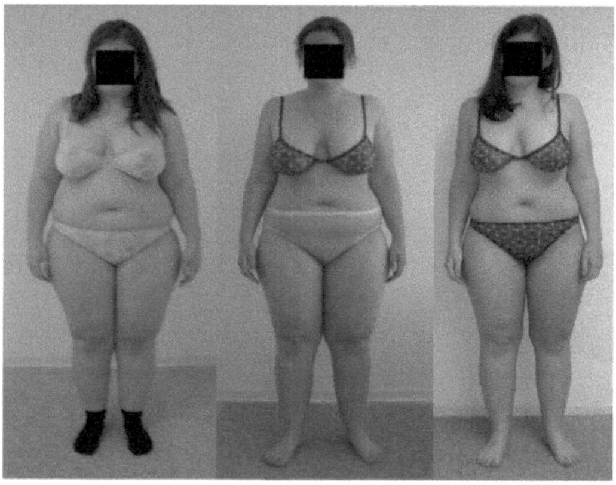

Figure 1

This case illustrates that Chinese medicine can help many patients with different indications.

## 2. Philosophy of Yin and Yang

What is CCM medicine? Chinese medicine is based on the theory of Yin and Yang. Let's take a closer look at this theory which was discovered in China. Nowadays everybody knows the words Yin and Yang, but their meaning is often fairly unclear.

Yin and Yang are basically the offspring of geographical observations and a deep understanding of the principles of nature. If you stand in the Northern hemisphere, facing South while watching the sunrise and sunset and the change between darkness and daylight, you will be able to observe the different aspects of the stars whose positions vary during spring, summer, autumn and winter. The Yin/Yang symbol and its development reflect these phenomena.

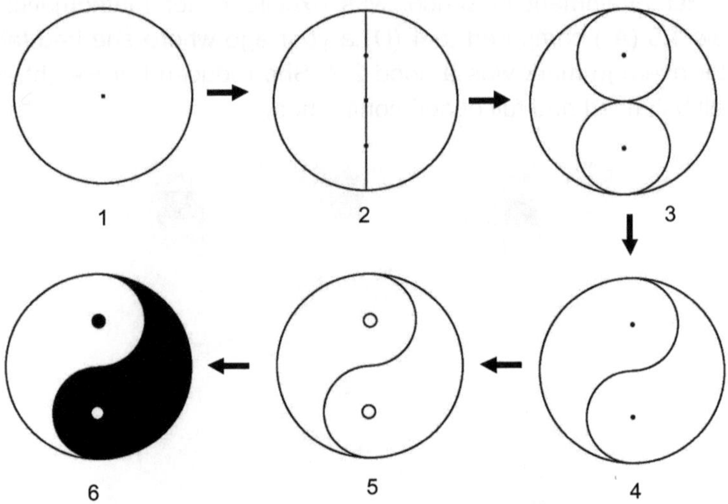


Figure 2

The sign stands for dynamic change. It contains as much information of the cosmos as can be comprised by a single symbol – the Yin/Yang symbol. The Yin/Yang symbol is more than just a symbol; it represents the general rules of our macrocosm:

1. Yin and Yang represents a system or content that has certain aspects. The content is embedded in a circle which has directions and borders, and is multidimensional. The circle changes its size according to the content.
2. The system contains two opposite pairs – Yin and Yang.
3. The Yin and Yang symbol is by no means a fixed image. It is permanently in motion and rotates in all directions.

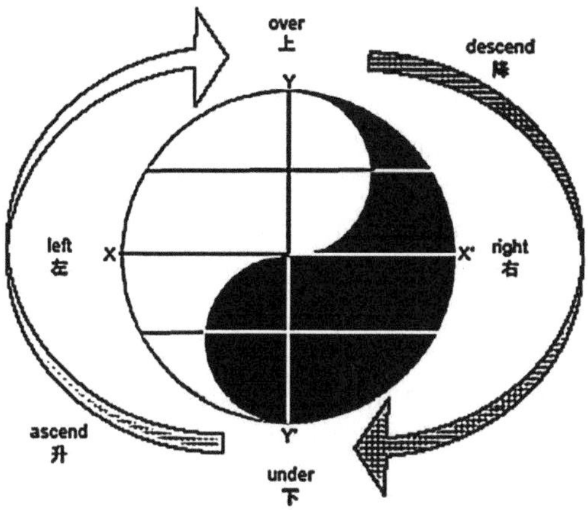


Figure 3

4. Movement implicates and requires time. The system starts at minimum, increases with time and inflates until it ends at the maximum point (y, y', Figure 4 a) where it transforms into the opposite. This goes on forever.

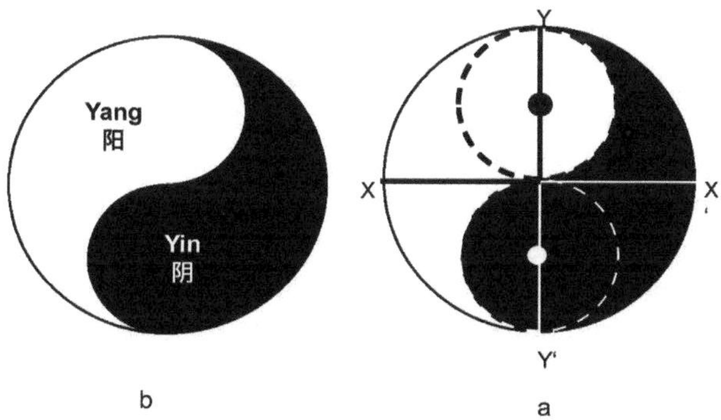


Figure 4a and 4b

5. Each black and white area changes its volume in the system, but its basic quality remains unchanged, i.e. black stays black and white stays white.
6. The system changes its quality whenever there is a transition from inflation to deflation and vice versa at a specific point in time (y, y') (Figure 4 b).
7. Under normal conditions the Yin and Yang symbol illustrates an imbalance which changes constantly. There is only one equilibrium point (x, x') that only lasts for a very short time. This is considered an absolute point.
8. The system can be broken down ad infinitum. This is symbolized by the different coloured point in each half.

The Yin/Yang symbol thus shows us a system which is dynamic and permanently changing. We live under and with this system. The terms "Yin" and "Yang" are abstract concepts which nevertheless can be explained further. The primary explanations of Yin and Yang are based on observations of the rhythm of day and night. Yin is characterized as "dark", "calm", "cold", "passive", "sinking" whereas Yang is characterized as "light", "warm", "active", "ascending". These four opposite pairs are only the basics of a sophisticated philosophy.

The Yin/Yang principle can be extended and fanned out to many more opposite pairs. The meteorological image depicting the four seasons also illustrates the Yin-Yang concept. It is a modern example of this principle that is applicable everywhere and which reminds us that everything is constantly changing and flowing as time passes. Yin elements are visible and palpable, e.g. anatomical structures, bones, muscles, nerves, blood, skin or inner organs. Although Yang elements are normally not visible and elusive they can be felt and measured. They work on the functional and energetic level, e.g. movement, body temperature, thought and speech processes, the functions of the inner organs, blood circulation and haematosis. When comparing Western and Chinese Medicine one might say that CCM is characterized by "Yang" and school medicine by "Yin".

Let's come back to the 8 principles mentioned above and illustrate them with some concrete examples to gather a better understanding as to how Yin and Yang function.

1. *Yin-Yang represents a system or content that has certain aspects. The content is embedded in a circle which has directions and borders, and is multidimensional. The circle changes its size according to the content.* School medicine mainly considers the human body, its organs and its pathological changes. CCM considers broader aspects, i.e. the individual, her living conditions and family, her job, the climate, influences from outside that effect the organ functions etc. When looking at the Yin and Yang symbol CCM works in a system that comprises many more aspects in such a circle than school medicine.

2. *The system contains two opposite pairs – Yin and Yang.* Our vegetative system is controlled through sympathicus (Yang) and parasympathicus (Yin). The sympathetic and parasympathetic systems show antagonistic results. Yet both, the sympathicus and parasympathicus regulate pulse rate, blood pressure or muscle tonus and fine-tune organ functions during stress and relaxation.

3. *The Yin and Yang symbol is by no means a fixed image. It is permanently in motion and rotates in all directions.*

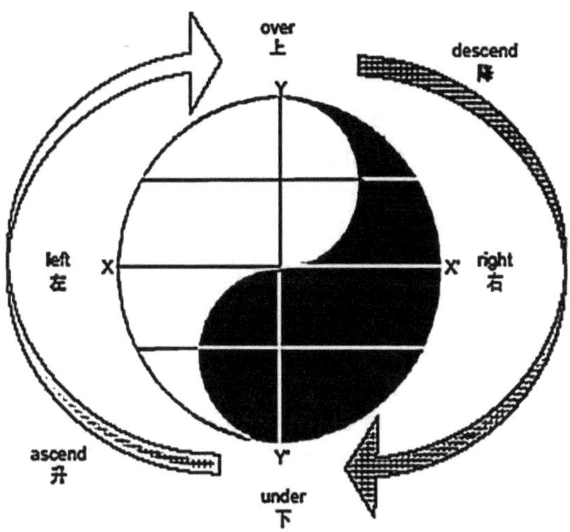


Figure 5

Every human being is dependent on his metabolism from birth to death. We know that every phase in life brings up specific problems which have to be taken into account during diagnosis and treatment. Every phase has a beginning and an end. Accordingly, a child requires a different treatment than an adult or an old person. Children are in an increasing Yang phase, adults are at the peak of the Yang phase, in their menopause/andropause men and women are in an increasing Yin phase, and seniors are at the peak of the Yin phase.

4. *Movement implicates and requires time. The system starts at minimum, increases with time and inflates until it ends at the maximum point (y, y', see Figure 4 a) where it transforms into the opposite. This goes on forever.* Our heart drives our life, the heartbeat works in the rhythm of time and depends on dilatation (Yin) and contraction (Yang). The phase of dilatation starts with a minimum of blood until it transforms into a phase of contraction. Each phase takes a certain amount of time until it reaches the tipping point. Normally the left heart chamber of an adult contains 120 ml of blood. When resting, 70 ml of blood are pumped out of the arteries during the systolic phase. Again, this takes time. This time and speed is reflected in the standard cardiac cycle of 60 to 80 heart beats per minute.

5. *Each black and white area changes its volume in the system, but its basic quality remains unchanged, i.e. black stays black and white stays white.* If there is a disorder our body sends a warning signal through the nerves, creating pain. But pain is not a disease. It is a symptom that indicates a physical disorder. Throbbing pain in the temple, for instance, is often caused by anger or stress and has a certain intensity that can be measured on a scale. The intensity of the pain might change, but if it still has the same quality the doctor will continue with the same treatment. The quality of pain and the area where it appears are decisive for therapy.

6. *The system changes its quality whenever there is a transition from inflation to deflation and vice versa at a specific point in time (y, y')* (see Figure 4 b). CCM therapy tries to regulate disharmony of Yin and Yang in the body. Pulse and tongue diagnosis determines the therapy which is modified as the disease changes. Let me illustrate this process with the flu. A distinct thick white coating on the tongue shows the beginning of this cold and is a symptom that the body is cold. As the body fights this coldness it develops inner heat until a yellow coating on the tongue develops. Thus, as the inner heat increases the body slowly reaches a tipping point

(y) where the white coating transforms into yellow coating. This is also the point where the nature of the flu changes and where therapy ends.

7. *Under normal conditions the Yin and Yang symbol illustrates an imbalance which changes constantly. There is only one equilibrium point (x, x') that only lasts for a very short time.* This is considered an absolute point. Our biorhythm works similarly because the human body is adapted to the rotating earth. Accordingly, cortical, insulin and hormone levels constantly rise and decline as they are synthesised and absorbed. Everything is in a constant flow. The state of our body also varies during day and night and with the seasons. Any equilibrium point that occurs is only a passing stage.

8. *The system can be broken down ad infinitum. This is symbolized by the different coloured point in each half.* Tissue can be broken down into cells, a cell broken down into chromosomes and other particles etc. This is the microcosm. The same applies to our earth, the planetary system, the galaxy and the universe, i.e. the macrocosm. The system can thus be extended in both directions. It is an open system, as is our body and organism. It has no hierarchy and all elements are subject to the same laws of the universe. Accordingly, the earth has a population of humans, which can be broken down into women and men. And women have male hormones as men have female hormones.

## 3. CCM medicine versus school medicine

CCM medicine and school medicine have very different approaches. The basics of both approaches are like a sprout that determines the result. Therefore I should like to analyse the main differences between these two philosophies. Let's take a closer look at the basic training.

### 3.1. The basics of CCM

CCM students start their basic training by learning three main principles:

1. Yin/Yang (philosophical background)
2. Jing-Luo (channels[1]) and Zang Fu (organ functions based on organ pairs)

---

1 I prefer the term "channel" to "meridians", as a meridian is two-dimensional, whereas a channel has three dimensions: depth, width and length.

3. Qi (effects of organ functions) and Xue (blood circulation and function)

The students train with a model that shows all the acupuncture holes[1] and positions of the channels. The mannequin is erect with both thumbs pointing forward and open palms towards the sides of the body. This basic posture illustrates the Yin/Yang positions, the pairs and opposites and that the channels are constantly circulating around the body. The future CCM doctor will automatically always have this circulating movement in his mind. Most important is the position with Yang parts on the top, the back, left and exterior side and Yin parts on the front side, right side and inner parts. The Jing-Luo system is translated with "channel". But there are no visible channels. It is only through Xué"穴 (translated as "hole") and the coincidence with different symptoms that we can recognize disorders and the regulation of disorders. The Jing-Luo system knows local holes synchronous to different times of the day. Qi 气 and Xuè 血 are circulating, connecting the whole body from head to the foot, from the inner organs to the skin and from the torso to the extremities.

By viewing the acupuncture puppet you can see the holes which are painted onto the body. As the channels cannot be seen, it is unknown how old Chinese medicine discovered these lines. There is an assumption that access and knowledge is gained during Qi Gong sessions. I also noticed during the many years of research in acupuncture that certain channels sometimes appear on the body of patients as a white or red line that is approximately 3mm thick and disappears after about 30 minutes. The main problem is the verifiability. Many scientists try to show proof of these channels and to solve the mystery, but so far Jing-Luo cannot be clearly proven with existing methods.

Since all bodily functions are interconnected via the energy flow through these channels a doctor might treat the toe of a patient, even if the patient has a problem with his eye. This is a holistic approach which is in stark contrast to school medicine where an ophthalmologist would concentrate solely on the eye and disregard the rest of the body. In the ancient

1 I prefer the term "hole" instead of "point", as the specific areas of the body for acupuncture are areas where it is particularly good to access the underlying stream of energy. As with "meridians", this translation from the Chinese is not quite correct and leads to many misunderstandings.

CCM scriptures the term "Qi" is omnipresent. It is at the core of the training and everything revolves around a person's state of Qi. What is Qi all about? The term "Qi" is very old, thus it is very difficult to describe. Different types of Qi serve to describe different states of the life force and vital functions. Qi is not palpable, nevertheless the doctor can tell in which state the patient's Qi is by looking at his eyes or tongue, by feeling his skin or by looking at his posture and aura. Qi is the result of manifold cell functions and the patient's physical state.

Basically, Qi is elusive and like a movement that constantly changes. Even if a person is sitting without motion Qi is still roaming about her body as the blood continues to flow, new cells are being created and the metabolism works. Qi shows the vital functions of a person and varies accordingly. Thus there is also weak Qi, Qi showing impending death and dead Qi. Over time anatomy was no longer important for CCM, as it worked almost exclusively with the sophisticated channel system and Qi. This means that CCM no longer dealt, for instance, with the size of an organ.

Another important concept in CCM is blood 血 (Xue). Blood is also very important for vital functions. The entire blood function is connected to the cardiovascular functions. Everything is about the heartbeat which is responsible for blood pressure and blood circulation. Blood carries oxygen. Only blood can circulate through the entire body and thus interconnects all the organs and cells. In the fetus the heart is the first organ to develop. This shows that blood is vital for life. Therefore, for Chinese Medicine the heart is the "emperor" which underscores the heart's significance. For this reason the tongue and pulse diagnosis was developed in order to assess the cardiovascular functions, i.e. blood flow (Yang) as well as its speed and the blood thickness. This means that even in ancient times CCM doctors were very well aware of the fact that blood is the driving force for life. Nevertheless, CCM doctors do not deal with changes in blood cells or organs. Instead they observe Qi and Xue to regulate the body accordingly.

## 3.2. The basics of school medicine

Now let's compare western medical school with CCM. In their first semester the students have anatomy lessons as basics. Anatomy is important because they learn everything about cells, tissues, organs and their functions in the human body. They also learn positions such as anterior, posterior etc. to describe organ positions but nothing about Ying /Yang aspects or channel pairs. Western medicine concentrates on isolated functions, but teaches nothing about energy flows and circulation.

On the other hand school medicine has excellent, sophisticated descriptions of cells, tissues and organs which are entirely lacking in CCM. The body is regarded as an object. This eventually produces a growing number of specialists for biopsies, kidneys, cardiovascular functions etc. Of course cardiologists also analyse cardiovascular functions, for instance, with the ECG. Nevertheless, school medicine still concentrates mainly on measuring and collecting anatomical information. School medicine applies special therapies when pains or dysfunctions have already occurred and prescribes drugs that have an effect on the deepest cellular level. Another area where school medicine excels is surgery which can save people's lives. The fields of oncology, orthopaedics (prostheses) and emergency medicine have also made great strides and can save lives. CCM medicine, in contrast, is often more effective when treating chronic diseases and can regulate the body such that it regains a healthy state.

After this short comparison one can draw the conclusion that school medicine concentrates solely on the anatomical body, technologies and devices and is thus characterized by the Yin principle. Chinese Medicine and Therapy are characterized by the Yang principle, as blood flow is a Yang function and thus stands for movement.

### 3.3. Methods of diagnosis

Regarding the different diagnostic methods of CCM and school medicine you can describe CCM as a macroscopic[1] method and school medicine as a microscopic method.

The CCM diagnosis starts by regarding and inspecting the patient: his stature, form, body language, colour of skin, motor behaviour. The inspection of the tongue needs only a few seconds. There you notice the general conditions of the blood circulation and its current state. Beside the eye inspection a Chinese medicine doctor uses his ears, nose and fingers

---

1 The term comes from the Greek "makro" which means "long" or "great", and "skopie", which means "regarding". In general we understand this as a method "to notice with the eyes".

as instruments for the diagnosis, without machines but with a lot of knowledge. One of the most important features in Chinese medicine is the flowing of Qi, the activity level of the human being. Chinese medicine has a completely different understanding of “disease” where “disease” is seen as an imbalance of the body's system and the flow of energy.

While CCM has a more macroscopic approach, modern school medicine works more along the lines of microscopy. It uses modern technology with x-rays, ultrasonic imaging, computer tomography, biopsy, histology or genetic engineering with detailed measurements and results. A biopsy, however, where the blood and chemical functions are analysed shows changes which had already occurred, it doesn’t show the actual condition of the cell, as the cell has been isolated from the body and is no longer embedded in the energy flow. Basically the cell has already started to wither away.

Both approaches collect data but draw different conclusions. Therefore they apply different therapies. One main difference between school medicine and CCM is that CCM has options to discover early dysfunctions (e.g. complexion, skin colour, fatigue without clear cause, painful areas which are identified with palptation) in the body which might indicate future problems.

## 4. Holistic methods

The factor “time” is a major element in Chinese medicine. It is not abstract, but connected with a position in space. Normally time is described with a line – but time is not a ruler. Each time period indicates space. Time and space are in permanent movement and are like a rotating, moving spiral. All creatures follow the rhythm of the system and have a kind of biological clock which synchronizes itself with the day and night cycle or other cycles. Human beings change along with the rotation of our earth. This is the base of the CCM organ clock which reflects the bio rhythm of the human body. All 12 channels of the body have special active times. Cortical levels, for instance, change over the course of a day. Cortisone starts to rise at midnight, reaches its peak during the morning and then declines again.

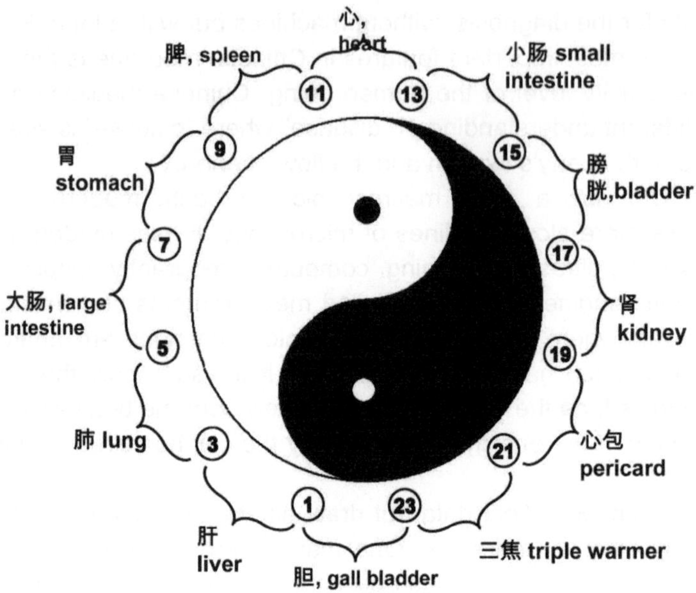


Figure 6

Scientific research looks for constant features and standards. It thus makes very much sense to carry out clinical trials to test the effectiveness of a drug for a specific group during a certain period of time. Individuals, however, cannot be treated according to such standard methods. Practical treatment needs a completely different approach. It has to take into account the complexity of the environment and time, regarding the individual patient and his or her life phase. Treatment has to be changed, adjusted or stopped according to the laws of nature. We need to observe these laws, otherwise we cannot be cured.

To find an adequate diagnosis, CCM takes into account the time frame when a disease breaks out, the daytime, the season, the age of the patient – all these factors play an important role. Every age group has special dysfunctions. The progression of a disease is also connected to time. In the beginning the disease shows minimal disorders, later these disorders are getting more and more evident. Healing with the help of a doctor or spontaneously also takes time. The earlier the disorder is recognized the earlier the condition can be healed. Chronic and severe diseases need longer therapeutic efforts in terms of time.

The environment where the patient is located plays a special role as every environment influences the human being. It's not really clear why epidemics occur at special places, special times and under certain circumstances. We know that certain diseases appear during very cold periods (about 2000 years ago) and other diseases appear during hot climatic periods (from 1400-1500). From the last century until now we have had a rise in allergies in many industrialized countries.

Our life sphere is a constantly changing system. Thus, individuals are also permanently changing. They are a microcosm reflecting the macrocosm. Therefore methods always have to be adapted to changing circumstances and one cannot repeat the same method as the quality of time and space and the patient's state will have changed until the next treatment is carried out. This brings me back to my original case. I treated the young lady according to her changing condition, based on the Chinese Yin and Yang principle. Since I always adapted therapy she recovered very quickly.

## 4. Conclusion

School medicine and CCM start off from different vantage points. This means, even though we observe the same object we derive different results and know only half of the story. The ultimate goal should be to join these two halves to create a greater whole.

A Chinese observer for instance, has different terms for the directions than a Western observer, because the Chinese sees himself as part of the earth that rotates. Thus the Chinese sees the sun is in front of him (South versus North for a Westerner) and his shadow behind him (North versus South for a Westerner). A Western astronomer regards the whole earth as an object that far away and not in relation to himself.

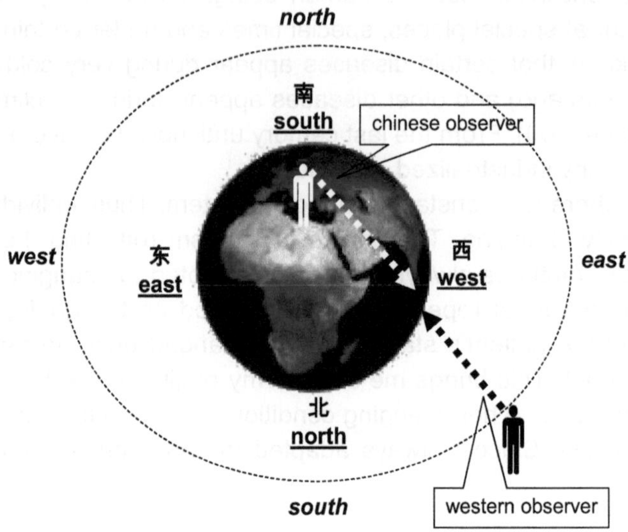


Figure 7

Based on their different approaches, East and West thus use different kinds of information given by their environment and have developed different methods regarding medicine, prophylaxis and medical treatment. It is not adequate to reject one system – the integration of both systems and other effective methods will lead medicine towards a general system. We need to learn to deal with hard and soft data. We need to learn that if we recognize a disorder, the next disorder might already be present. If a disease doesn't develop in a typical way, it is often not discovered and treated. This means that a lot of time is lost. The earlier a diagnosis can be given, the more time is gained. Therefore, an early diagnosis is one of the most important postulations in our 21st century.

Gerhard Litscher

# High-Tech Acupuncture: A Successful Transcontinental Approach in Traditional Chinese Medicine

Abstract: Within the past century the scientific and technological progress has truly revolutionized Eastern and Western experimental and clinical medicine. This century was certainly the most innovative phase in medical history. Our research group has made various efforts within the last 13 years to modernize acupuncture [1-10], one of the most spectacular of Eastern medical procedures. For this reason we have developed and scientifically investigated new stimulation and measurement methods for quantifying the effects of acupuncture and moxibustion. For the application of stimuli at the acupoints we use manual needle acupuncture, laserneedle acupuncture and electrical methods. The usage of advanced exploratory tools such as multidirectional transcranial Doppler ultrasound sonography, cerebral near infrared spectroscopy, functional magnetic resonance imaging, different bioelectrical methods and other highly sophisticated biomedical equipment, provides revealing insights. The obtained results are absolutely necessary for the acceptance of acupuncture by the Western medical community. Goal of this contribution is to present new possible study designs for the evidence of specific effects of acupuncture in the periphery and the brain (cross-over studies). In addition, first double-blind studies in acupuncture research using painless laserneedles and first transcontinental multi-center studies [11] in this area of modern research will be presented.

## Introduction

With the help of newly developed helmet constructions and with complex high-tech neuromonitoring equipment it was possible for the first time to provide evidence of cerebral functional changes during acupuncture. Since 1997 the Research Unit of Biomedical Engineering in Anesthesia and Intensive Care Medicine of Graz Medical University has been dealing with the demystification of acupuncture and examining, using non-invasive methods, how different stimulation modalities (manual needle acupuncture, laser acupuncture, electro acupuncture) affect central and peripheral functions.

In this chapter, the first medical data in acupuncture research obtained with a violet (blue) laser beam will be presented [12]. This kind of laser is new and has only been used in industrial applications (blu-ray disc). There are no published data available in medical acupuncture yet (www.pubmed.gov).

Moxibustion is an Asian healing method, which is able to achieve specific warming effects at special acupoints. The effects of a new Japanese needle-moxa-system were evaluated in a transcontinental three-center pilot study in Graz, Beijing and Seoul using high-tech measuring methods.

The heart rate variability (HRV) and especially the LF/HF ratio become more and more important as a specific indicator for a well-balanced autonomic nervous system in different disciplines of medicine. Acupuncture and acupressure seem to have positive effects on these parameters and the proper function of the autonomic nervous system (ANS) [7]. The main purpose of a randomized cross-over pilot study was to investigate the specific effects of acupuncture and acupressure on the mean heart rate, the HRV and particularly on the LF/HF ratio.

Telecommunication technology includes the assisted transmission of signals and biological data over a distance. In this context telemedicine like telesurgery and also teleanesthesiology have become more interesting. However, teleacupuncture has not yet been performed [12].

The patients' and doctors' interest in acupuncture has grown dramatically in Western society in the past decade. The increased use of acupuncture is attributed to its medical efficiency, cost effectiveness and credibility provided by clinical trials and biomedical research. In this context a lot of new innovative medical devices have been developed and experimentally investigated in Austria at our research institution recently.

Methods

Using complex multidirectional ultrasound examinations evidence of cerebral functional changes after acupuncture could be provided for the first time (Fig. 1).

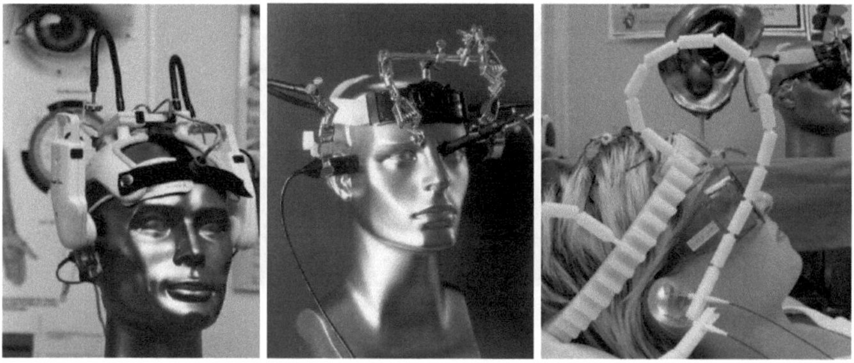

Fig. 1: Multifunctional helmet constructions for acupuncture research (mod. from [12]).

Many people nowadays are fascinated by the term laser. Innovation and laser have nearly become synonyms. Laser is also an important instrument for acupuncture. One only needs to mention the treatment of children or of patients with needle phobia. In this way individual combinations of acupuncture points can be stimulated simultaneously according to TCM. In the context of double-blind studies (neither the acupuncturist nor the patient knew whether the stimulation was activated or deactivated) effects in the brain could be demonstrated in a reproducible manner for the first time.

The aim of a study presented in this paper was to investigate specific temperature and microcirculation effects of blue/violet laser acupuncture by stimulating the acupoint Hegu (LI.4), using a continuous beam. The changes of temperature and blood circulation were quantified in the area around this acupoint (distance: 1 mm) and at the fingertip of the index finger before, during and after stimulation in 15 healthy volunteers (mean age: 27.9 ± 5.6 years, range 22 – 35 years; 11 f, 4 m) using infrared thermal imaging (Flir i5, Flir Systems Inc., Portland, USA) and a laser Doppler system (DRT4, Moor Instruments Ltd., Devon, UK). Painless violet laser light (wavelength: 405 nm; output power: 110 mW; diameter: 500 µm, activation: 10 min) was used (Fig. 2) [12].

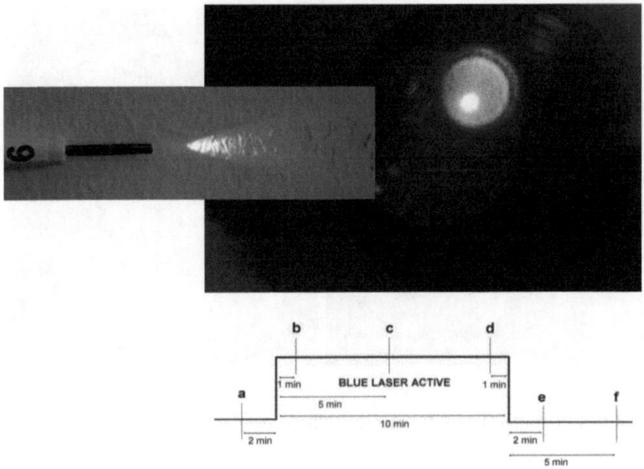


Fig. 2: Non-invasive violet laser acupuncture stimulation and measurement procedure (modified from [12]).

Concerning the new moxibustion system (Fig. 3), basic technical temperature measurements were performed in Seoul. In addition, nine investigations were carried out in six healthy volunteers (3 f, 3 m; mean age: 27.2 ± 5.7 years) using different methods (thermography, laser Doppler flowmetry, laser Doppler imaging and heart rate variability). Four persons were examined in Graz, two in Beijing. Moxibustion was always applied at acupoint CV 6 (Qihai). In addition, biosignal registrations were carried out in Graz during painless laser acupuncture of acupoint CV 12 (Zhongwan).
In the context of a medical traineeship at the Beijing University of Chinese Medicine twenty-five healthy volunteers (12 f, 13 m; mean age ± SD: 26.5 ± 8.6 years) underwent three procedures consisting of acupuncture on extrapoint 1 (Yintang), acupressure on the same point and placebo acupuncture at a sham point over 10 minutes. The sequence of the three methods was randomized. All volunteers were monitored over a period of 20 minutes using an electrocardiogram recorder (Medilog AR12). The data before, during and after the three conditions were measured and statistically analyzed.

In the first teleacupuncture pilot study worldwide, 24-hour ECG (electrocardiogram) recordings performed at the China Academy of Chinese

Medical Sciences in Beijing are presented [12]. The ECG was recorded with a sampling rate of 4096 Hz using a system partially developed in Austria (medilog AR 12, Huntleigh Healthcare, Cardiff, UK). The raw data were transferred via internet to the TCM Research Center Graz in Austria from the patients' site computer in Beijing to the control site computer in Graz (distance: 7,650 km). Data analysis of different parameters of heart rate (HR) and heart rate variability (HRV) in the time and frequency domain [7] was performed immediately for control of possible therapeutic effects of acupuncture. The acupuncturist and the monitoring expert were informed about the findings immediately and the success of the therapy could be demonstrated objectively.

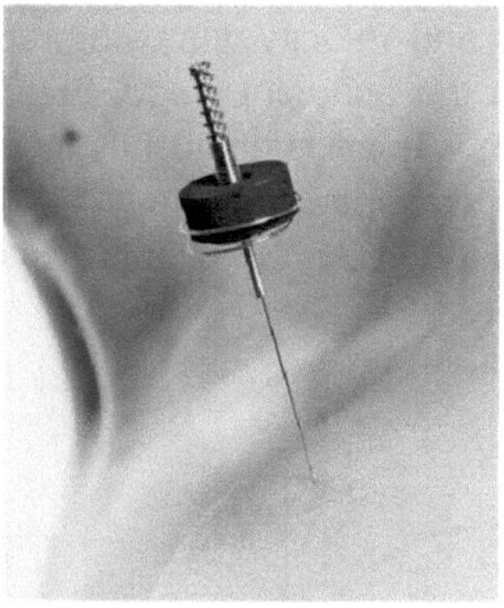

Fig. 3: A new system for acupuncture moxibustion.

The electrical punctual stimulation system (P-Stim) reflects a new, miniaturized high-tech system for pain therapy and stress reduction through ear acupuncture [13]. Ultrathin needles were applied at special ear acupoints. In February 2009, 24-hour measurements were performed at the Beijing University of Chinese Medicine by an Austrian researcher (M.K.) in close cooperation with Chinese medical doctors using this new medical electrical stimulation equipment. Ten healthy Chinese volunteers (5 f, 5 m; mean age ± SD: 24.8 ± 1.9 years; range: 21-27 years) were investigated. To evaluate the different opinions concerning the new system a questionnaire in both English and Chinese language was created. The persons were given this questionnaire after the 24-hour measurement.

Results

The stimulation of acupuncture points, which according to traditional Chinese medicine (TCM) are to improve vision, led for example to an increased blood flow velocity in the ophthalmic artery. Apart from the blood flow velocity the regional cerebral oxygen saturation also changed. The stimulation of points which according to TCM are to increase brain function generally leads to a significant increase in the flow velocity of the middle cerebral artery.

First investigations of the violet laser stimulation yielded interesting results. Ninety percent of the subjects felt the stimulation performed on the acupoint similar to deQi-sensation. There were significant increases in temperature ($p \leq 0.001$; paired t-test) and Flux ($p \leq 0.001$), which is the product of concentration and velocity of moving red blood cells, during violet laser acupuncture at the acupoint Hegu. Five minutes after acupuncture, Flux at this location was still significantly increased ($p \leq 0.001$), temperature showed values similar to baseline ($p = 0.185$, n.s.). There was no significant effect in temperature and Flux at the tip of the index finger [12].

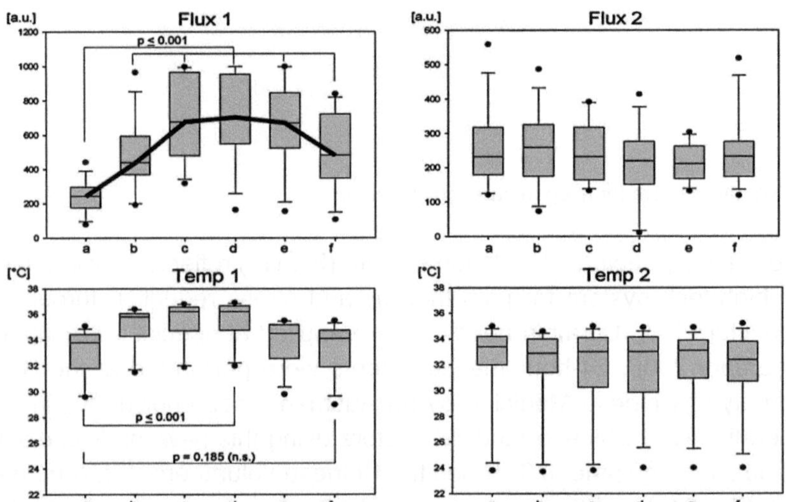


Fig. 4: Changes in Flux (= product of concentration and velocity of erythrocytes) and temperature 1 mm beside Hegu (LI.4; Flux1, Temp1) and at the tip of the index finger (Flux2, Temp2). Note the significant increase in microcirculation (Flux1) during acupuncture (comp. Fig. 2). Modified from [12].

During moxibustion, temperature distributions and changes in microcirculation (at isolated spots and as a large-area image) were registered. The dimensions of local and temporal effects of heat stimulation can be visualized objectively (Fig. 5).

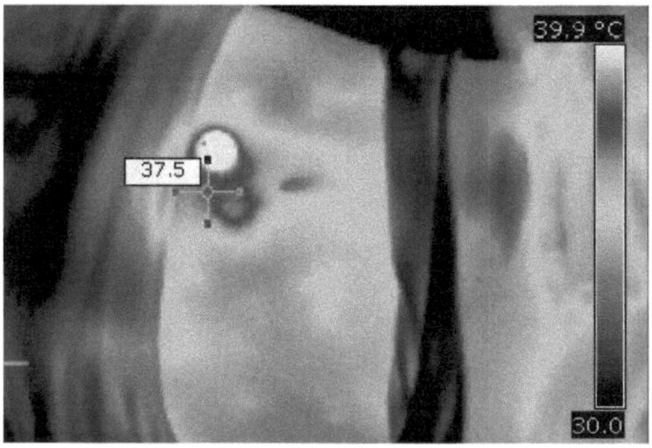


Fig. 5: Temperature value during moxibustion in a 21-year-old female volunteer. The picture shows scaling on the right and the actual temperature value on the left at the particular measurement point. Modified from [14].

The study of heart rate variability during stimulation at the acupoint Yintang showed the following results: The mean heart rate values decreased significantly during verum acupuncture and acupressure on Yintang ($p \leq 0.001$). The changes during acupuncture on the sham point were also significant ($p = 0.002$). Acupressure reduced the LF/HF ratio in all volunteers noticeably. A division into gender showed that the LF/HF ratio tended to decrease in both groups, but especially the females showed an obvious reduction of the LF/HF ratio during and after acupressure.

It was the aim of a biomedical pilot measurement to investigate whether teleacupuncture using computer-controlled HRV analysis can be performed over long distances (transcontinentally) using common internet connections (Fig. 6). As modern internet connections allow a transfer with more than 100 Mbit/s, even the real online transfer of a high-resolution ECG signal with an adequate sampling rate should not be a problem in the future [12].

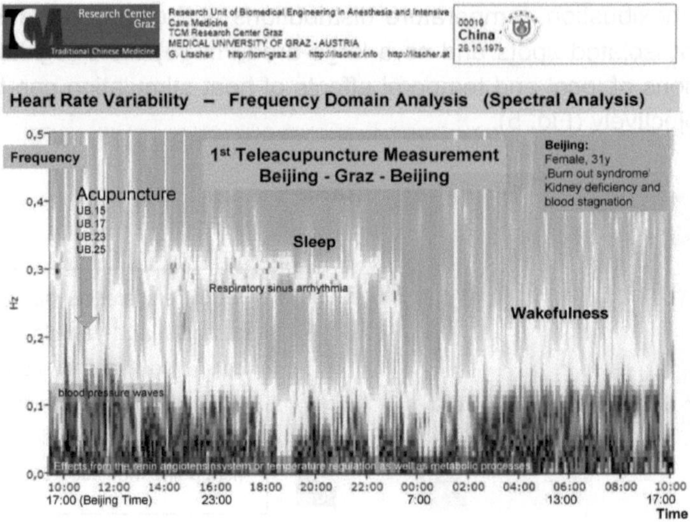


Fig. 6: First teleacupuncture measurement between Graz and Beijing (modified from [12]).

The results of the punctual electrical long-term stimulation show that most students felt better after treatment and were relaxed during and after treatment (very good 10 %, good 30 %, satisfactory 60 %, poor 0 % and very poor 0 %). A typical statement from a Chinese student (C.B., 21 y) was: *"During treatment I feel a little nervous. But in the evening I sleep well. Thanks for the good machine."*

## Discussion and Conclusion

With new biomedical technology constructions and technical monitoring procedures, which comprise amongst others light, ultrasound and highly sensitive bioelectrical measuring processes, it is possible for the first time to demonstrate reproducible specific effects of laser acupuncture both peripherally and centrally.

Blue laser light with a wavelength of 405 nm which appears to the eye as violet may represent a new approach to high-tech acupuncture research. First results are promising as shown in this manuscript. Further studies using this new kind of technology in medical research are absolutely necessary.

Effects of the new moxibustion method can be quantified reliably by modern measuring equipment. Using this system, moxibustion under standardized conditions can now be performed with a minimum of smoke emission and a high degree of safety [14].

From the heart rate variability measurements we concluded that acupuncture but especially acupressure reduced the LF/HF ratio. This effect was more pronounced in females and could be interpreted as an expression of growing vagal activity during acupressure [15].

The first realization of teleacupuncture demonstrates that automated teletherapeutic procedures can be performed even over a long distance (7,650 km) under complex and critical circumstances. This could probably be useful under special circumstances, e.g. in case of a cooperation between experts from different continents [12].

The questionnaire in context with the electrical punctual stimulation system demonstrated that most students (60 %) experience only little pain when the needles were applied. Electroacupuncture using P-Stim seems to be a method which according to the patients' perception has a positive influence on their state of health. Further investigations are in progress.

Acknowledgements
The following scientists delivered valuable contributions to this manuscript: Weibo Zhang (Beijing, China), Seung-Ho Yi (Seoul, Korea), Lu Wang (Graz, Austria), Tao Huang (Beijing, China), Ingrid Gaischek (Graz, Austria), Yu Ying Tian (Beijing, China), Guangjun Wang (Beijing, China), Verena Ganglbauer (Graz, Austria), Zheng Xie (Beijing, China, and Graz, Austria), Yi-Jun Wang (Beijing, China), Baixiao Zhao (Beijing, China), Jan Valentini (Beijing, China, and Graz, Austria), Martina Kollmann (Graz, Austria). The author wishes to thank everyone sincerely.

The studies were supported by the Zukunftsfonds Styria (project 4071). The investigations are part of the project "Bioengineering and clinical assessment of high-tech acupuncture – a Sino-Austrian research pilot study", supported by the Federal Ministries of Science and Research and of Health and the Eurasia Pacific Uninet.

References

1. Litscher G. Bioengineering assessment of acupuncture, part 1: thermography. Crit Rev Biomed Eng 2006; 34(1):1-22
2. Litscher G. Bioengineering assessment of acupuncture, part 2: monitoring of microcirculation. Crit Rev Biomed Eng 2006; 34(4):273-294
3. Litscher G. Bioengineering assessment of acupuncture, part 3: ultrasound. Crit Rev Biomed Eng 2006;34(4):295-326
4. Litscher G. Bioengineering assessment of acupuncture, part 4: functional magnetic resonance imaging. Crit Rev Biomed Eng 2006; 34(4):327-345
5. Litscher G. Bioengineering assessment of acupuncture, part 5: cerebral near infrared spectroscopy. Crit Rev Biomed Eng 2006; 34(6):439-457
6. Litscher G. Bioengineering assessment of acupuncture, part 6: monitoring – neurophysiology. Crit Rev Biomed Eng 2007; 35(1):1-38
7. Litscher G. Bioengineering assessment of acupuncture, part 7: heart rate variability. Crit Rev Biomed Eng 2007; 35(3):183-195
8. Litscher G. Ten years evidence based high-tech acupuncture – a short review of peripherally measured effects. eCAM 2007; DOI 10.1093/ecam/nem145
9. Litscher G. Ten years evidence based high-tech acupuncture – a short review of centrally measured effects. eCAM 2007; DOI 10.1093/ecam/nem169
10. Litscher G. Ten years evidence-based high-tech acupuncture, part 3: A short review of animal experiments. eCAM 2008; DOI 10.1093/ecam/nen034
11. Zhang WB, Wang LL, Huang T, Tian YY, Xu YH, Wang L, Litscher G. Laser Doppler perfusion imaging for assessment of skin blood perfusion after acupuncture. Medical Acupuncture 2008; 20(2):109-118.
12. Litscher G. Modernization of traditional acupuncture using multimodal computer-based high-tech methods. J Acupunct Meridian Stud 2009; 2(3): 202-209.
13. Széles JC, Litscher G. Objectivation of cerebral effects with a new continuous electrical auricular stimulation technique for pain management. Neurol Res 2004; 26:797-800.
14. Litscher G, Zhang WB, Yi SH, Wang L, Huang T, Gaischek I, Tian YY, Wang GJ. The future of acupuncture moxibustion: a transcontinental three-center pilot study using high-tech methods. Medical Acupuncture 2009; 21(2):115-121.
15. Litscher G. Effects of acupressure, manual acupuncture and Laserneedle acupuncture on EEG bispectral index (BIS) and spectral edge frequency (SEF) in healthy volunteers. Europ J Anaesthesiol 2004; 21:13-19.

Fengli Lan

# Metaphorizing: A Vital Way to Understand and Modernize Chinese Herbal Medicine

The formulation of most of the books on Chinese materia medica has been almost fixed in the writing pattern of "Properties, Flavors, Channels Entered, Actions, Cautions & Contraindications" since the era of *Shennong's Classic of Materia Medica*, but few explain or illustrate whys and hows.[1] The Chinese herbal medicine, just like Chinese medicine, has evolved under the guidance of *Tian Ren He Yi* 天人合一 or Universe and Man Uniting and Resembling Each Other through *Qu-Xiang Bi-Lei* 取象比类 or Taking Image and Reasoning from Analogy.

## 1. *Qu-xiang Bi-lei:* the Metaphorizing Process in Chinese Herbal Medicine

*Qu-xiang Bi-lei* can be summarized into four steps as stated in *The Book of Changes*: 1) Observing objects or phenomena (*guan wu* 观物): directly observing objects or phenomena; 2) Taking image (*qu xiang* 取象): summarizing and refining the image of the object or phenomenon after repeatedly observing and feeling it; 3) Comparing and analogizing (*bi lei* 比类): comparing the things which need to know with the "image (*xiang* 象)"; 4) Understanding the Way or Rule (*ti dao* 体道): finding the rules. The whole process ends in the formation of metaphors. Therefore, *Qu-xiang Bi-lei* can be regarded as the metaphorizing process, is a vital methodology to understand and research Chinese herbal medicine, and plays a vital role in constructing and developing Chinese herbal medicine.

1 LING Yikui. Textbook for Medical Higher Education (5th Edition): Chinese Herbal Medicine [M]. Shanghai: Shanghai Scientific and Technical Publishers, 1984: 1.

## 2. Metaphorizing: A Vital Way to Understand Chinese Herbal Medicine

"To truly modernize Chinese medicine, we must first demystify these theories." (Wang Ming-wei)[1]

### 2.1 Differences between *Ben Cao* and *Yao*

It is well known that Chinese medicine uses mixtures of different medicinal substances formulated according to a certain strategy in a holistic approach to disease. Here first of all, I would like to discuss the differences between *Ben Cao* (Materia Medica, 本草) and *Yao* (Medicine, 药).

*Ben Cao* (Materia Medica, 本草) and *Yao* (Medicine, 药) have been taken as the same since the teaching mode of Chinese medicine has transformed into the modernized or Westernized or professional one at the early of the 20th century. That is to say, *Yao* is a modernized term of *Ben Cao.* Actually, they do not refer to the same thing.

*Ben Cao*, the materia medica, is a collective term for all of the individual substances with healing properties, i.e. the medicinal substances or the medicinals, including herbs, minerals and animal parts. *Ben Cao* is divided into three grades in the *Shennong's Classic of Materia Medica*:

- Top-grade medicinal: is non-toxic, possesses a rejuvenating effect and can be taken frequently and for a long period of time without causing any harm;
- Medium-grade medicinal: has no or only slight toxic effect and is effective in treating diseases or supplementing deficiencies;
- Low-grade medicinal: is effective in expelling pathogens, but is toxic and should not be taken for a long period of time.

*Yao,* 藥, its original Chinese character, is explained to be "harmony of different medicinal substances", and is used to "treat illnesses" (the character is 疒 with 樂 inside it, a variant form of 療, the simplified character is 疗), i.e. restoring the harmonious state to the individual. The two characters of the original forms share the same part 樂 (the simplified form is 乐, means music, is explained to be "harmony of different tones" in *The Origin of Chinese Characters*. Thus, it is clear that *Yao* 藥 refers to the medicine ready to be taken for treating illnesses, which is usually composed of more than

1 QIU, Jane. China Plans to Modernize Traditional Medicine [J]. Nature, April 2007: 590-591.

one medicinal substance formulated according to the strategies of *Jun Chen Zuo Shi* or Chief, Associate, Assistant and Guide medicinals, i.e. formula. I think the Chinese Herbal Medicine is composed of the two parts: *Ben Cao* (Materia Medica, 本草) and *Yao* (Medicine made from a Formula, 药).

## 2.2 Metaphorizing: A Vital Way to Understand Materia Medica (*Ben Cao*)

### 2.2.1 Theory of Chinese Materia Medica Comes from Metaphorizing Qi, Yin-Yang and Five Phases

Everything in the universe, including Man and Chinese Materia Medica, comes into being by the movement and mutation of Qi, which begets Yin-Yang, and the five phases (two pairs of yin and yang, i.e. water and fire & wood and metal, plus one middle soil).

*The Four Properties* (si qi, 四气) result from metaphorizing the Yin-Yang of the Heaven, varying according to the four seasons – Warm and Hot, the Yang of the Heaven; Cool and Cold, the Yin of the Heaven. In specific, properties of a medicinal come from metaphorizing its living environment, growing seasons and rules, collecting time, and/or medicinal part (including its shape, color, etc.), etc.

*The Five Flavors* (wu wei, 五味) result from metaphorizing the Yin-Yang of the Earth, varying according to the five phases – Acrid, Sweet, and Bland, the Yang of the Earth; Sour, Bitter, and Salty, the Yin of the Earth. It is well know that flavors of many medicinals are far away from their real tastes.

*The Channel Entry* (gui jing, 归经) results from attributing the medicinal's properties and flavors to Man's *zang-fu* organs according to the theories of Yin-Yang and Five Phases.

### 2.2.2 Metaphorizing: A Vital Way for Genesis of Actions of Materia Medica

*Tian Ren He Yi* or Universe and Man Uniting and Resembling Each Other is the philosophical foundation for metaphorizings of Chinese Materia Medica, and metaphorizing is the way to know the actions of Chinese medicinals, which of course have been confirmed and proved in the clinical practice.

Actions of a Chinese medicinal are from metaphorizing its property, or its flavor, or its color, or its shape, or its quality, or its disposition, or its growing time, or its growing place, etc. which is used to harmonize the *zang-fu* organs and restore Yin-Yang balance to the individual with its predominating actions.

*Metaphorizing Its Property:* Cool or cold medicinals have the actions of clearing heat, draining fire, cooling blood and reducing toxicity, etc; while warm or hot medicinals have the actions of warming the interior, dispersing cold, supplementing fire, reinforcing yang, warming the channels and freeing the network vessels, restoring yang from collapse, etc.

*Metaphorizing Its Flavour:* Generally speaking, acrid medicinals can disperse and promote the flow of qi and blood; sweet can tonify, moderate, and harmonize; sour can astringe; bitter can drain fire and dry dampness; salty can soften the hardness and free the bowels; bland can promote urination, etc.

*Metaphorizing Its Colour:* Such a viewpoint has been systematized and theorized by the aid of the five-phase theory since the Han dynasty (206B.C.-220A.D.). *Essentials of Materia Medica* (Ben Cao Bei Yao . Yao Xing Zong Yi) states that the medicinals of green-blue with sour taste pertains to wood, all enter the Liver and Gallbladder Channels (The liver stands interior-exterior relationship with the gallbladder, the gallbladder is Jia wood, the liver is Yi wood); that of red with bitter taste pertains to fire, all enter the Heart and Small Intestine Channels (The heart stands interior-exterior relationship with the small intestine, the small intestine is Bing fire, the heart is Ding fire) ; that of yellow with sweet taste pertains to earth, all enter the Spleen and Stomach Channels (The spleen stands interior-exterior relationship with the stomach, the stomach is Wu earth, the spleen is Ji earth); that of white with acrid taste pertains to metal, all enter the Lung and Large Intestine Channels (The lung stands interior-exterior relationship with the large intestine, the large intestine is Geng metal, the lung is Xin metal); that of black with salty taste pertains to water, all enter the Kidney and the Bladder Channels (the kidney stands interior-exterior relationship with the bladder, the bladder is Ren water, the kidney is Gui water.). [Note: Jia, Yi, Bing, Ding, Wu, Ji, Geng, Xin, Ren, Gui: the ten heavenly stems.]

For example: There are five colours of beans to enter the five zang organs respectively. Black bean, black in color, its shape is like that of the kidney, the grain of the kidney, so can tonify the kidney; Red bean, red in color, the grain of the heart, with downbearing property, can free the small intestine and has the function of diuresis; the white hyacinth bean, white and yellowish, the grain of the spleen, can regulate the spleen and warm the stomach. The following are some other examples illustrated with pictures.

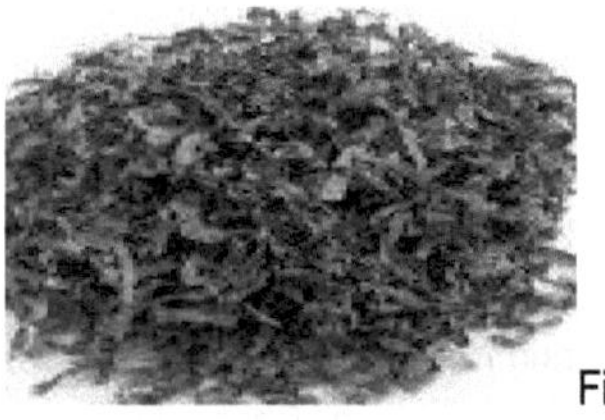

Fig.1 Sang Ye

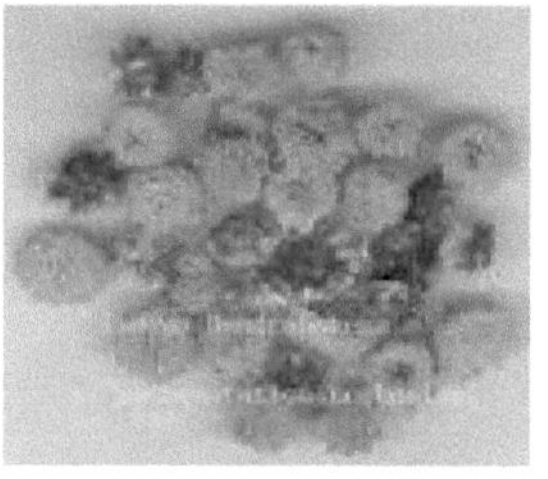

Fig.2 Ju Hua

The greenish, whitish, yellowish medicinals are usually said to enter the phase of *qi*, used to treat exterior pattern, such as mulberry leaf (Folium Mori, Sang Ye; Fig.1) and chrysanthemum (Flos Chrysanthemi, Ju Hua; Fig.2)

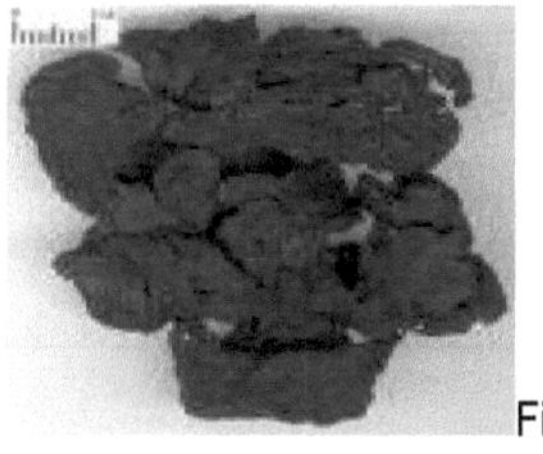

Fig.3 Di Huang

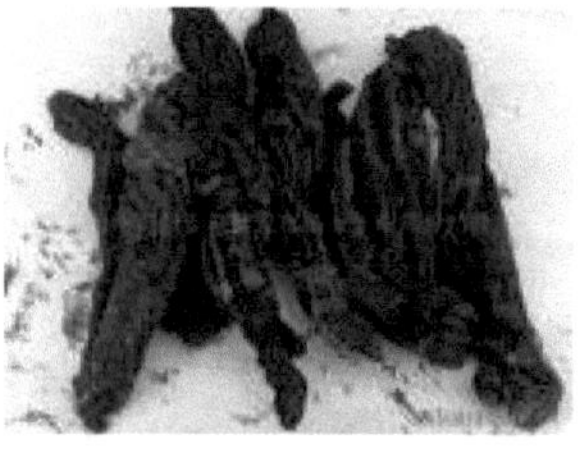

Fig.4 Xuan Shen

The reddish, blackish, dark yellow medicinals are usually said to enter the phase of blood, used to treat interior pattern, such as rehmannia (Radix Rehmanniae, Di Huang; Fig.3) and scrophularia (Radix Scrophulariae, Xuan Shen; Fig.4).

Besides, green-blue, red, yellow, white and black medicinals are attributed to different zang-fu organs according to the five-phase theory. For example:

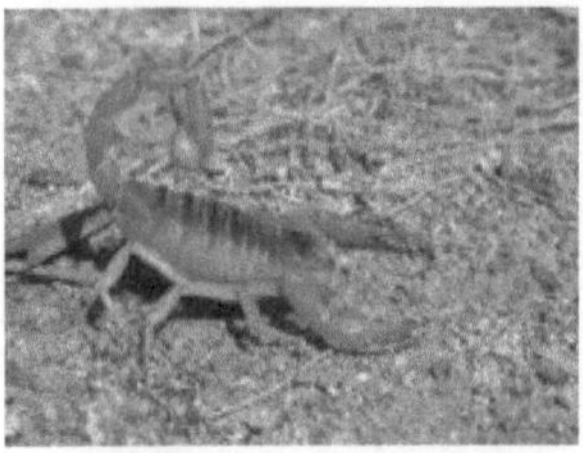

*Scorpion* (Buthus, Quan Xie, Fig 5), whose body colour is *green-blue*, is said to enter the *Liver* Channel, and is therefore used to treat *wind disease*, such as convulsion, spasm, stubborn bi syndrome (such as arthritis), etc.

Fig.5 Quan Xie

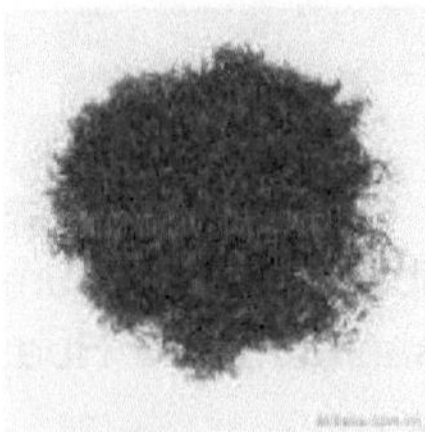

*Carthamus* (Flos Carthami, Hong Hua, Fig.6), whose colour is *red*, is said to enter the *Heart and Liver* Channels, and therefore is used to promote the flow of blood, remove blood stasis, and free menstruation for the *blood* is from the heart and is stored in the liver.

Fig.6 Hong Hua

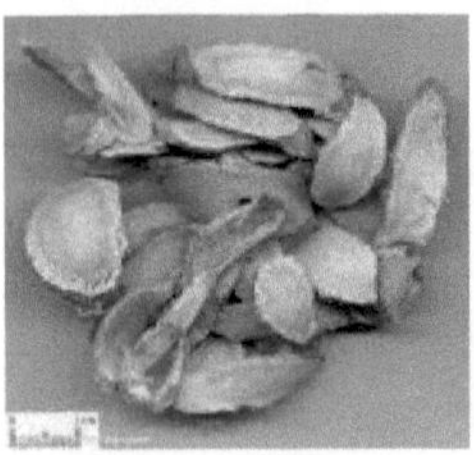

*Astragalus* (Radix Astragali, Huang Qi, Fig.7), whose colour is *yellow* and whose flavour is *sweet*, is said to enter the *Spleen* Channel, and is therefore very effective in *tonifying the Spleen and benefiting Qi.*

Fig.7 Huang Qi

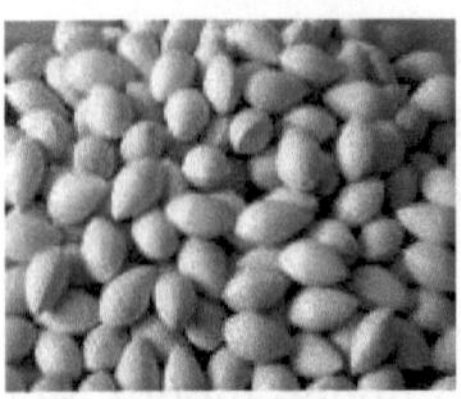

*Gingko* (Yin Xing, Fig.8), whose colour is *white*, is said to enter the *Lung* Channel, and is therefore used to supplement the Lung Qi and arrest coughing.

Fig.8 Yin Xing

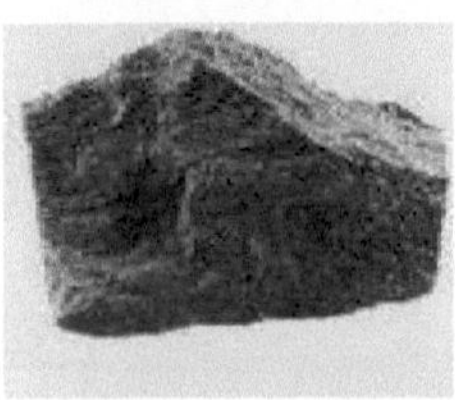

*Magnetite* (Ci Shi, Fig.9), whose colour is *black* and *heavy* in quality, is said to enter the *Kidney* Channel, and is therefore used to tonify the Kidney and subdue yang, arrest panting, deafness and tinnitus caused by Kidney deficiency, downbear the reverse upward flow of Qi.

Fig.9 Ci Shi

Some medicinals with more than one colour or even five colours can be used to treat various diseases. For example, Jujube is formed from small white flower to fruit of first green, then white and yellow, then red after being ripe, then blackish after being picked up and dried under the sun, bearing the colours and qualities of the five phases, and therefore can nourish the Spleen and Stomach, free and open the nine orifices, benefit the twelve channels, supplement qi, engender fluid, tonify the blood, supplement deficiencies of all kinds, harmonize all of the other medicinals, etc. (Zhang Zhi-cong, Ben Cao Chong Yuan or *The Origin of Materia Medica* . Ben Jing Shang Pin or Top Grade Medicinals of *Shennong's Classic of Materia Medica*)

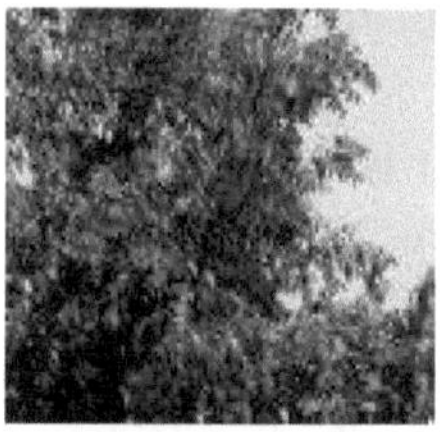

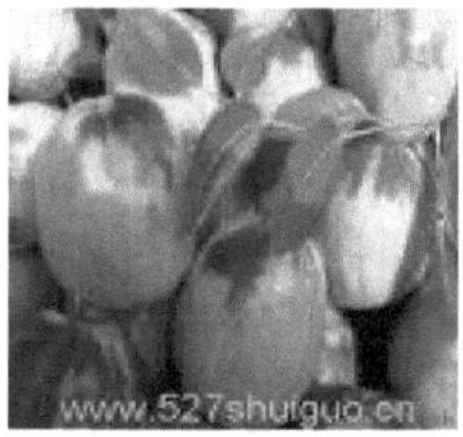


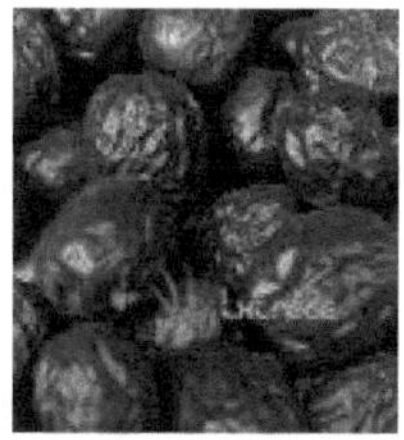

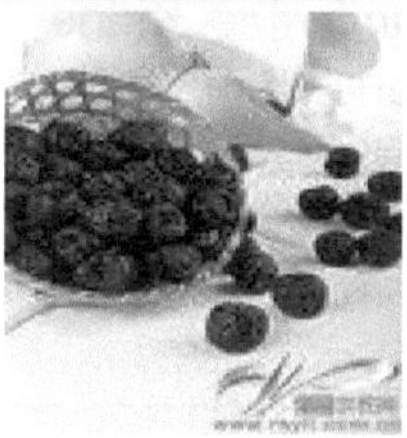

Fig.10 Jujube (Chinese Date, Da Zao)

*Metaphorizing Its Shape:* The typical example is ginseng. The Chinese name is Ren Shen 人参, of which Ren 人 means human being. Zhang Zhi-Cong's *The Origin of Materia Medica* (Ben Cao Chong Yuan . Ben Jing Shang Pin) states that the root of ginseng is like the shape of the human being with head, face, and the four limbs. It receives the brilliance of the Heaven and the vastness and richness of the Earth, and forms into the shape of the human being after a long time, thus having the quality of the Heaven, Earth, and human being. Therefore, it is mainly indicated in supplementing or tonifying the human being.

Besides, ginseng mainly grows in the damp shadow places of forests in the North-East of China, can survive in one of the world coldest places, and is therefore very effective in restoring yang from collapse and contraindicated in excessive and heat patterns, such as the famous Pure Ginseng Decoction (Du Shen Tang).

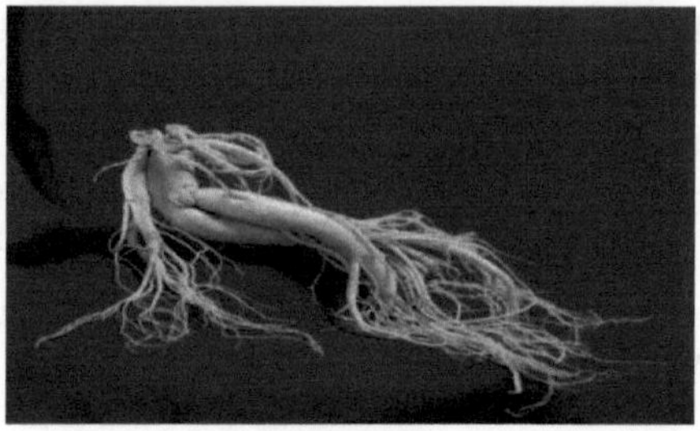

Fig.11 Ginseng

*Metaphorizing Its Disposition:* Generally speaking, flower is usually on the tip of a branch, and therefore can expel the pathogenic factors on the head and eyes; the leaves distribute around a plant in different directions, and therefore can disperse; stem and branch can treat diseases of the limbs; seed conceives a new life, and therefore can tonify the Kidney, strengthen sexuality, help conceiving a fetus, and treat sterility or infertility; hollow medicinals or with holes can free the flow of qi and free the network vessels; medicinals rich in fluid can increase humour; vine can free the network vessels; and so and so forth. Take krait for example.

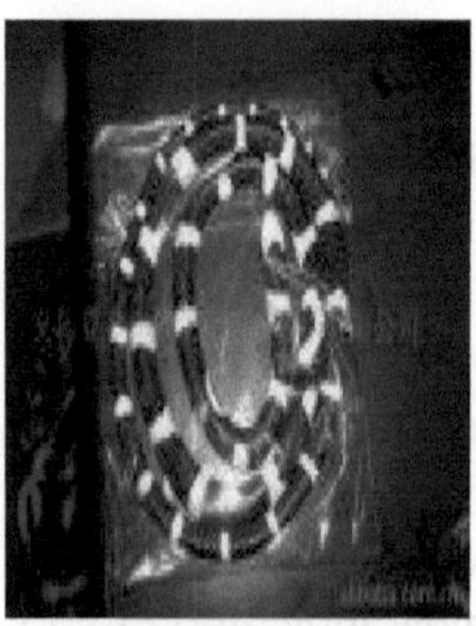

Fig.12 Krait

"The snake can treat all kinds of wind diseases. ... The wind moves swiftly and is changeable. The snake also moves swiftly and exuviates (casts off or sheds) many times in its life. Therefore, it can track wind deep into the bone, stabilize convulsions (caused by wind), and is an important medicinal for wind blockage disease, convulsions, leprosy, tinea, serious sores and ulcers for it can move through the bowels and viscera inside, run through the skin outside, can reach nowhere in the body". (Li Shi-Zhen, Ben Cao Gang Mu or *The Compendium of Materia Medica*)

Take seeds as another example. *"The seed (籽) can produce semen* （子） ". *Shen Nong's Classic of Materia Medica* read that Wu Wei Zi (schisandra, Schisandrae Fructus) can benefit or supplement the male's semen; *A Collection of Annotations on Classic of Materia Medica* (Ben Cao Jing Ji Zhu) states that Gou Qi Zi (lycium berry, Lycii Fructus) can tonify essential qi, strengthen sexuality; *On Properties of Medicinals* (Yao Xing Lun) records that Tu Si Zi (cuscuta, Cuscutae Semen) can benefit essence or semen and supplement marrow, and that Fu Pen Zi (rubus, Rubi Fructus) is indicated in deficiency or depletion of kidney essence for the male and infertility for the female; *A Collection of Words on Materia Medica* (Ben Cao Hui Yan) states that Che Qian Zi (plantago seed, Plantaginis Semen) can strengthen sexuality and help conceiving a fetus; and so and so forth. A version of textbook "*Chinese Herbal Medicine*" published in the 1950's states that "most of the medicinals rich in seed are said to enter the kidney", and we know that kidney is responsible for growth, development and reproduction in Chinese medicine. There are some formulae which are mainly composed of different seeds, such as Seven-Seed Powder recorded in the *Invaluable Prescriptions for Emergencies* (Bei Ji Qian Jin Yao Fang) mainly for male's sterility due to deficiency of essential qi, Five-Seed Progeny Pill recorded in *Introduction to Medicine* (Yi Xue Ru Men) as "the No.1 prescription for conceiving a fetus of all times", and Pill of Five-Seed and Whole Deer recorded in *The Black Bead in the Red Water* (Chi Shui Xuan Zhu) for sterility due to yang deficiency.

To sum up, all of the Chinese medicinals come into being and shape from the Qi of the Heaven and Earth, have different actions, and therefore can treat different illnesses, which can be inferred from metaphorizing their qi (property), flavour, colour, shape, quality, etc. through *Qu-Xiang Bi-Lei* outlined in the framework of *Tian Ren He Yi*.

### 2.3 Metaphorizing: A Vital Way to Understand Medicine made from a Formula (*Yao*)

It is a great qualitative leap of the development of Chinese herbal medicine from single medicinal to a formula, in which therapeutic interactions among different medicinals are strengthened, while toxicity or side effect is reduced through coordinated action of different medicinals. To identify the pattern and establish a treating principle is the premise of prescribing a formula, which is generally composed of Chief, Associate, Assistant and

Guide medicinals, a holistic approach to disease treatment of harmonizing different aspects of the patient:

- *Sovereign [Chief]:* provides the principal therapeutic action;
- *Minister [Associate]*: helps strengthen the principal action;
- *Adjuvant [Assistant]*: relieves secondary symptoms or tempers the action of the Chief when the latter is too potent;
- *Courier [Guide]*: directs action to the affected channel or site.

3. Metaphorizing: A Vital Way to Modernize the Chinese Herbal Medicine

Previous attempts to modernize Chinese herbal medicine have focused on isolating active ingredients from the herbal remedies and screening them one at a time, which accords with the Western way of thinking, i.e. analytical or abstract thinking. And such an approach has led to a handful of new treatments, such as artemisinin for treating malaria and the decongestant ephedrine, "but there has been no goldrush of approved drugs." The Western way of thinking can be an ideal complement to the Chinese way of thinking, and the corresponding research outcome provides valuable references for both researchers and practitioners. But I think the Chinese way of thinking should be of more significance in guiding the studies on modernizing Chinese herbal medicine.

*The 1st Example – Tripterygium Wilfrodis* (Lei Gong Teng 雷公藤)[1]: Li Leishi 黎磊石 discovered for the first time the therapeutic effect of Tripterygium Wilfrodis in treating various chronic nephritis, lupus nephritis, and purpuric nephritis, and spread it to the whole country through metaphorizing Tripterygium Wilfrodis's immunosuppressive action in taking effect in treating nephritis and allergic dermatological diseases. Later on he proved the effect of an ingredient isolated from this herb in acute rejection after renal transplantation, and clarified Tripterygium Wilfrodis's immunosuppressive action in an all round way.

1 LI Leishi. Personal Experiences in Integrating Chinese Medicine with Western Medicine [J]. Chinese Journal of Integrated Traditional and Western Medicine, 1998, 18 (12):707.

*The 2nd Example – Realgar-Indigo Naturalis Formula* (RIF, Fu Fang Qing Dai Wan, 复方青黛丸)[1]: The main components of RIF are realgar (xiong huang, 雄黄), *Indigo naturalis* (qing dai, 青黛) and *Salvia miltiorrhiza* (dan shen, 丹参) with tetraarsenic tetrasulfide (A), indirubin (I), and tanshinone IIA (T) as their major active ingredients respectively. The research group took the active ingredients as the representatives of the three medicinals (a kind of metaphorizing) to study the synergy in the treatment of a murine APL model *in vivo* and in the induction of APL cell differentiation *in vitro*. Their data also indicate A as the principal component of the formula, whereas T and I serve as adjuvant ingredients. They therefore suggest that dissecting the mode of action of clinically effective formulae at the molecular, cellular, and organism levels may be a good strategy in exploring the value of traditional medicine. This case has been regarded as a successful case of researching compound formulas of Chinese medicine. Therefore, the strategy of composing a formula (Chief, Associate, Assistant and Guide medicinals) will be a valuable strategy in discovering or synthesizing new drugs. [2]

To sum up, I think metaphorizing is a vital way to understand, to research, to and modernize Chinese herbal medicine, and will be also a valuable strategy in discovering or synthesizing new drugs.

---

1 WANG Lan, ZHOU Guang-Biao, LIU Ping, et al.. Dissection of Mechanisms of Chinese Medicinal Formula Realgar-Indigo Naturalis as An Effective Treatment for Promyelocytic Leukemia [J]. PNAS (Proceedings of the National Academy of Sciences of the United States of America), 2008, Vol. 125 (12): 4826-4831.

2 QIU, Jane. 'Back to the future' for Chinese herbal medicines [J]. Nature, 2007 (6): 506-507.

Jianguo Qin, Yahong Wang, Zhangan Jin, Shuoren Wang, Weiqin Guo

# Effect of Jiangzhi Tongmai Fang on Regulating the Expression of Liver Basal Membrane Heparan Sulfate Proteoglycan in ApoE-knock-out Atherosclerosis Mice

Abstract: *Objective* To observe the effect of Jiangzhi Tongmai Fang (JZTMF) on regulating expression of liver basal membrane heparin sulfate proteoglycan in ApoE-knock-out atherosclerosis mice. *Methods* Wild type group: 12 C57/BL mice were fed common diet for 90 days. 36 Apoe-knock-out mice were fed a Western-type diet for 90 days and were randomized into three groups: model group, JZTMF group and Simvastatin group. For wild type group and model group, 0.9% normal saline was given. For JZTMF group and Simvastatin group, JZTMF or Simvastatin were given. TG, TC, LDL-C and HDL-C were measured by the end of experiment. The expression of liver basal membrane heparan sulfate proteoglycan (HSPG) was analyzed by immunoblot. *Results* JZTMF and Simvastatin reduce level of serum total cholesterol and low density lipoprotein, up-regulate expression of liver HSPG when mice were fed with high fat diet, but improve level of serum total cholesterol and low density lipoprotein and down-regulate HSPG expression, compared with wild type group fed with common diet. *Conclusion* JZTMF reduces serum cholesterol and low-density lipoprotein level and up-regulates HSPG expression in ApoE-knock-out mice. Up-regulation of HSPG expression is one of mechanisms to prevent and cure atherosclerosis.

## Introduction

Atherosclerosis (AS) is the basic pathological change of cardiac, cerebral and vascular diseases. The basic methods to reduce morbidity and death resulted from cardiac, cerebral and vascular diseases are to prevent or ameliorate AS. JZTMF is used for improving function of spleen and removing phlegm and blood stasis and clinically effects well on hyperlipemia and atherosclerosis. Using animal, we want to know how JZTMF regulates serum lipids and liver basal membrane heparin sulfate proteoglycan (HSPG) of C57/BL-ApoE-knock-out mice.

1. Materials and Methods

1.1 Animal

Eight weeks old healthy male C57/BL-ApoE-knock-out mice and wild type C57/BL mice were maintained in Animal Institute, Health Science Center, Beijing University.

1.2 Medicine

JZTMF is made from Rensheng, Zexie, and so on? It is given by Professor Peigen Xiao of Beijing Chinese Medicine University. Simvastatin (or named Shujiangzhi, P1076) was made by MSD, Hangzhou, China.

1.3 Animal model and groups

Mice were divided into four groups. Wild type control group: C57/BL fed with common diet and undergone lavage with 0.9% physiological saline. Model group: C57/BL-ApoE knock-out mice fed with high-fat diet (0.15% cholesterol, 21% fat, Beijing Granule Keao Ltd. Co.) and undergone lavage with 0.9% physiological saline. JZTMF group: diet as model group, but undergone lavage with JZTMF. Simvastatin group: diet like model group, but undergone lavage with Simvastatin. The medicine dose applied to mice is 10 times of that applied to human and the concentration is 10 g/mL. Medicine were applied to mice once a day, continuously for 90 days.

1.4 Serum lipids measurement

After 90 days' medicine administration, mice were treated with limosis for 12h, then performed anaesthesia with 3% chloral hydrate. 1 mL blood was collected from aorta abdominalis, centrifuged at 2000 rpm for 15 min and serum was harvested. Using kits (from Beijing Lideman Biochemical Technique Limited Corporation) to measure total serum cholesterol (TC), glycerin trilaurate (TG), high density lipoprotein (HDL) and low density lipoprotein (LDL).

1.5 Western blot to check HSPG expression

After 90 days' medicine administration, mice were treated with limosis for 12h, then anaesthesia with 3% chloral hydrate. Livers were collected and homogenized at 4°C, centrifuged at 16,000g, 4°C for 15min, then the supernatant was harvested. Total protein concentration was measured by Lorry's method.

Using 50 ug total protein for SDS-PAGE, hemi-dry-transferred to nitrocellulose membrane (NC), blocked with 5% milk/TBS overnight at 4°C. NC membrane was washed with TBS thrice, then applied with anti-HSPG (in 5% milk/TBS and 0.05% tween-20), overnight at 4°C. Washed with TBS thrice, NC membrane was applied with alkaline phosphatase-labeled secondary antibody (in 5% milk/TBS) overnight at 4°C. Washed with TBS thrice, NC membrane was developed by chemiluminesence. Data were processed with Alpha imager 2200 (Alpha Innotech Co., USA) and Quantity One 6.0 (Bio-Rad Laboratory) software.

### 1.6 Statistics

Serum lipids data were shown as mean ± sd and analyzed by ANOVA. HSPG expression bands were shown by values of photodensity as mean ± sd and values of mean were compared.

## 2. Result

### 2.1 Change of serum lipids

Serum TC value of JZTMF group is less than that of model group and the value of Simvastatin group is much lower than that of model group. LDL values of JZTMF group and Simvastatin group are much lower than that of model group. There is no apparent difference for HDL among groups. Data are shown in Table 1.

Table 1 Concentration of serum lipids (mean ± sd, mmol/L)

| Group | n | TC | TG | HDL | LDL |
|---|---|---|---|---|---|
| JZTMF | 8 | 13.61±1.83** | 1.71±0.61 | 2.03±0.39 | 8.00±2.32*** |
| Simvastatin | 8 | 13.24±2.04*** | 1.59±0.86 | 2.21±0.09 | 9.27±1.55*** |
| Model | 8 | 17.21±1.38 | 1.83±0.77 | 2.25±0.09 | 14.37±1.34 |
| Wild type control | 8 | 1.61±0.32 | 0.52±0.26 | 1.27±0.39 | 0.17±0.06 |

**, $p < 0.01$; ***, $p < 0.001$, compared to model group.

### 2.2 Expression of HSPG in liver basal membrane

HSPG expression in liver basal membrane of model group is down-regulated, compared to that of wild type control group. HSPG expressions of JZTMF group and Simvastatin group are up-regulated, compared to that of model group, but down-regulated compared to that of wild type control group. Data are shown in Figure 1 and Table 2.

Figure 1. Expression of HSPG in groups

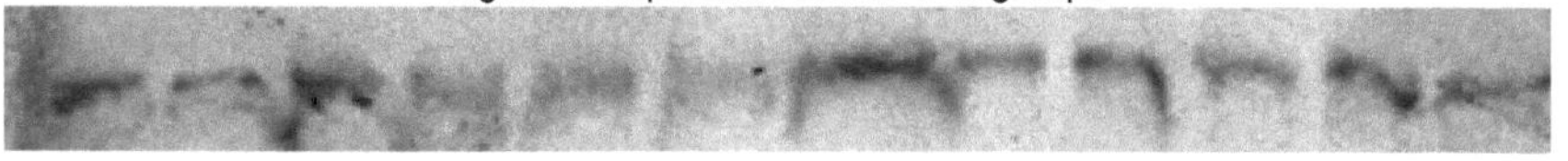


1、2、3 Con. G , 4、5、6 Mod. G , 7、8、9 JZTMF G , 10、11 、12Simvastatin G

Table 2: Optical density of liver basal membrane HSPG expression bands (mean±sd)

| Group | Photodensity |
|---|---|
| JZTMF | 130.00±28.05 |
| Simvastatin | 122.67±11.53 |
| Model | 87.00±14.17 |
| Wild type control | 147.00±37.98 |

## 3. Discussion

In liver, chylomicron remnants (CMR) are removed by low density lipoprotein (LDL) receptors of hepatocytes, or by receptors coordinated with LDL related protein (LRP) and HSPG on cell surface, or directly by HSPG. CMRs are mainly removed in liver while proteoglycan is also involved in this procedure. Proteoglycan exists on surface of liver endothelial cells and supplies with hepatic lipase and lipoprotein lipase. In Disse chamber, heparin sulfate proteoglycan binds hepatic lipase and Apoe. After CMRs enter this chamber, it is modified by hepatic lipase and Apoe that are heparin binding proteins. Disse chamber can reserve and filter CMRs before they are absorbed by hepatocyes. It is reported that the proteoglycan mainly exists in Disse chamber and lipoprotein is absorbed at the same location where proteoglycan exists in liver. It is also reported that, in diabetes mice, clearing of Apoe-48 lipoprotein delays. Serum cholesterol and LDL levels increase because liver basal membrane HSPG expression decreases. So HSPG has very important role in metabolism of blood lipid and formation of atherosclerosis.

We created atherosclerosis model by feeding ApoE-knock-out mice with high fat diet. ApoE-knock-out mice can form severe hyperlipidemia and AS focus whatever it is fed with normal or high fat diet. And it becomes good model to study pathogenesis and intervening treatment of hyperliemia and AS. Sunny H Zhang found that plasma total cholesterol (TC) level of Apoe-knock-out mice fed with normal diet is about 5 times of that of normal mice. Because we used high fat diet to create animal model, plasma TC level is about 10 times of normal animal, higher than that was reported. It is possibly related to high fat diet.

Simvastatin, is an inhibitor of HMG-CoA reductase. HMG-CoA reductase is rate-limiting enzyme in procedure of cholesterol biosynthesis. By specific competition, Simvastatin inhibits HMG-CoA reductase and methyldihydroxypentanoic acid cannot form, and cholesterol level decreases. JZTMF and Simvastatin's failure to bring down triglyceride level indicates that high blood lipid level is closely related to diet insobriety. Medicine cannot control it well.

Weiqin Guo reported that atherosclerosis is related to diet insobriety, over-taking fat and sweet food, too much rest, less exercise and aging. Atherosclerosis forms because spleen and kidney become deficient, phlegm and blood stasis impede obstruction of meridians. High blood lipid level is the key of AS. High blood lipids are phlegms and spleen is the source of phlegms. If spleen does not work well and dysfunctions, nutrition cannot be absorbed normally, then phlegm and blood stasis occurs and blood lipid level surges and it promotes atherosclerosis. The formation of atherosclerosis is a long procedure and it frequently happens to the middle age, so renal deficiency is the key point. The dysfunction of spleen, kidney and other internal organs is the basic element of AS. Their transferring ability loses and phlegm forms, or Qi becomes deficient and cannot be diffused, blood stops flowing and silts. "Medicine master must read—Tanyin" tells us when spleen becomes deficient, the clean does not go up and the dirt cannot deposit. Something stops in the chest and phlegm forms. "Yiguan—Tanyin" tells us kidney deficiency cannot control water and water cannot go to the source. If water goes wrong way and flood will happen and phlegm will occur. The formation of blood stasis and turbid phlegm is because Qi and blood become deficient in chest, they interact and jam the vessel, then atherosclerosis occurs. The author suggested that we should shape spleen, tonify kidney, minimize phlegm and dredge vessel and these are basic rules to treat atherosclerosis. The author created the recipe of JZTMF, which contains Renshen and Zexie. Renshen is bitter, mild and good for heart, lung and spleen. Renshen can supply Yuanqi, make lung and spleen healthier, create saliva and calm nerves. "Benjing" tells us that Renshen can make five internal organs healthier, calm nerves and remove pathogenic factors. "Function of Medicine" tells us Renshen is in charge of deficiency of five internal organs, five fatigues and seven injuries. "Rules to Use Medicine" tells us that Renshen is sweet and mild, and can supply Yuanqi in the lung. If Yuanqi becomes strong, Qi in the four internal organs will be strong, energy will happen spontaneously and the body will be powerful. It is because the lung is in charge of every Qi. It is reported that saponin in Renshen can apparently reduce TC, TG and LPO level in blood of mice with high fat diet. Zexie is sweet, dilute, cold and helpful to kidney and bladder. It makes water and heat permeate easily. "Benjing" also tells us that Zexie is in charge of chill and moist, secret milk, permeate water and ameliorate five internal organs and energy. "Bencao Gangmu" tells us Zexie can permeate moist and heat, reduce phlegm. "Bencao Zengyi" tells us that Zexie can reduce phlegm. Phlegm accumulates water and moist and becomes pathogenic. If phlegm is smooth, then it will be reduced. It is reported that Zexie is anti-oxidant, regulates lipid metabolism and prevents atherosclerosis.

The data indicate that JZTMF strengthens spleen, removes phlegm and dredges vessel, and it also reduces level of TC, LDL in serum of atherosclerosis Apoe-knock-out mice induced by high fat diet. It also regulates HSPG expression of liver basal membrane. This is basic study of JZTMF that regulates HSPG and it need further study in order to reveal the mechanism of strengthening spleen, removing phlegm and dredging vessel to prevent atherosclerosis. We hope this to be a guide to clinical practice.

## References

Yahong Wang, Mingjing Zhao, Xiyin Lu, et al. Study of JZTMF's effects on hyperlipemia and atherosclerosis. Journal of University of Beijing Chinese Medicine. 2001, 24 (3):20-24

Yahong Wang, Weiqin Guo, Suoren Wang, et al. The effect of JZTMF-treated serum on vascular endothelial cell. Journal of Chinese Medicine. 2004, 19(10):601-603

Plump A S, Jonathan D Smith, Tony Hayek, et al. Severe hypercholesterolemia and atherosclerosis in apolipoprotein E-deficient mice created by homologous recombination in ES. Cell. 1992, 71 (10): 343-353

Sunny H Zhang, Reddick R L, Piedrahita J A, et al. Spontaneous hypercholesterolemia and artherial lesions in mice lacking apolipoprotein E. Science. 1992, 258 (10):468-471

S O Kolset and M Salmivirta. Cell surface heparin sulfate proteoglycans and lipoprotein metabolism. Cellular and Molecular Life Science. 1999, 56:857-870

Park L, et al. Suppression of accelerated diabetic artherosclerosis by the solubal rceptor for advanced glycation end products. Nat. Med. 1998, 4:1025-1031

Tetsu Ebara and Karin Conde. Delayed catabolism of Apoe-48 lipoproteins due to decreased heparin sulfate proteoglycan production in diabetic mice. J Clin Invest. 2000, 105 (12) 1807-1818

Yunxiang Fang, Zhousheng Xiao. Renshen total saponin regulates serum lipids of mice with high fat diet. Journal of Hunan Medical University. 1995, 20(5):425

Hongfei Si, Ping Xiang, Likun Yang, et al. Study of Zexia and Lentinus edodes' function of anti-oxidation and regulating serum lipids.

Friedrich G. Wallner and Fengli Lan

# Researching Chinese Medicine: Methods and Problems

Our work has the goal and the core to save Chinese medicine in the times of globalization because we think Chinese medicine will perish if it can not communicate with Western science. We say "communicate" because Western science has a totally different structure and totally different methods from Chinese medicine. Therefore the traditional Western philosophy of science cannot understand Chinese medicine and cannot explain Chinese medicine. The paper has three chapters: (1.) the difference between construction and description in respect to Chinese medicine, (2.) the function of metaphor in the structure of Chinese medicine – with some examples, and (3.) the difference between explaining and understanding in respect to Chinese medicine.

## 1. The difference between construction and description in respect to Chinese Medicine

### 1.1 Backgrounds of Western science: Stict division between theory and practice and construct of subjectivity

Now we show you the background of Western science in a new point and then we will go to the point: "Why Chinese science is overwhelming the Western science"? Western science has two important backgrounds which are only cultural convictions, which do not come from the nature somehow. The one is the strict division between theory and practice, theory and action, and the other one is the construct of subjectivity.

According to the first aspect – strict division between theory and practice – the Western medicine is an applied science. Chinese medicine is not an applied science, but a practical science, which pays much more attention to practical knowledge which aims to prevent and cure illnesses not the knowledge which mainly aims to understand the human body. This is an important difference.

But at this point we want to make you aware about a wrong way of interpretation we find sometimes in China and out of China. Chinese medicine is interpreted as a type of dialectics, something which can be referred to the dialectics of Hegel and Marx. This is the half-truth. It has something true in it because Hegel and Marx had already shown before me that the Western science is always suppressing the action, is always underestimating the human activity, and thus always underestimating the human subjectivity.

An interesting point of Marxism is the critics of Western science but not at all have they understood Chinese medicine. Last year we have shown already the function of subjectivity in the Western science. It is the Western way of thinking to *reduce the subject* in scientific work. It is the claim to take out your subjectivity from the object. Instead the Chinese way of thinking is based on a *unification of the subject and object.*[1] Subjectivity is a European invention in the times of the Greek thinking. Subjectivity is totally ununderstandable in the horizon of Chinese thinking. In the times of the Greek thinking they invented this dichotomy between the nature and the man, the object and the subject. And this dichotomy goes through all the European thinking until today. You can make a choice between Western Philosophers: if they point out, if they underline more the side of object or the side of subject. But the Western science was always eager to totally take the subjectivity out of its concept. Therefore the goal of Western science has been until today to describe the world as if there would be no describing persons, to describe the world as if there would be no observer. As soon as you become aware that there is always an observer – otherwise the description has no sense – then the Western sciene gets into troubles. These troubles we have in physics with the Quantum Theory – we cannot say if something is a particle or a wave. And System Theory was an important beginning to overcome this trouble. System theory is for me an important new start in the Western thinking started around 70 years ago.

We want to make you aware about a discussion which is very strong in the last years and now in Europe, the discussion about the consciousness and the free will from the point of view of neuroscience. We cannot discuss it in details here because this would be a full lecture, and it is not so easy to explain, but some neuroscientists' point of view is that they be-

---

1 Wallner, Friedrich. Five Lectures on the Foundations of TCM [M]. Frankfurt am Main: Peter Lang, 2009: 27-34.

lieve that they have shown, that they have proved that free will is impossible. But what we want to make you understand here is just this interesting mistake of the Western science in this point. They show that something is not existing what they have taken out beforehand. If you take out subjectivity, you cannot speak about free will. It is not needed to deliver a type of argumentation against free will. This is an interesting artifact.

### 1.2 Presupposition of Chinese Medicine: *TIAN REN HE YI*

In difference to these ideas Chinese thinking is totally different and – as you know – in Chinese thinking we have the basis on the pressuposition of the unity of living systems and world. Therefore – as you know – for Chinese medicine, astrology can also some times at least play a role and we would defend it that they use astrology because they have another framework than Western science. For the Western science astrology is a way of suspicious and doubtful thinking, they must exclude this reference; but the Chinese thinking has this reference from the living system to the whole world. Therefore, astrology – the movement of the stars – can be important.

In Chinese medicine, the Doctrine of Five Periods (wu yun, 五运) and Six Qi (liu qi, 六气) is aimed to interprete influences of movements of celestial bodies and climatic changes on the living systems by applying the dynamic rhythms of the five periods and six qi as well as transformation between and integration of them. We would like to give you an interesting example – outbreak of encephalitis B in Shijiazhuang, Beijing, and Guangzhou. In 1956, encephalitis B was prevalent in Shijiazhuang, Hebei province. White Tiger Decoction (bai hu tang, 白虎汤) formulated by Zhang Zhong-Jing (张仲景) was administered to patients, and the achieved therapeutic effects surpassed the world levels although no theories on microorganisms have ever existed in Chinese medicine; In 1957, encephalitis B was prevalent in Beijing. But the White Tiger Decoction did not yield notable effects. Pu Fu-Zhou (蒲辅周), a prominent physician in Beijing, added Rhizoma Atractylodis (cang zhu, 苍术) to eliminate dampness according to the doctrine of five periods and six qi, which achieved 90% rate of efficiency; In 1968, encephalitis B was prevalent in Guangzhou, Guangdong province. Deng Tie-Tao (邓铁涛), a prominent physician, identified the cause of the disease as summer-heat with latent dampness according to this doctrine, and gave patients corresponding prescriptions based on pattern identification, which achieved 90% rate of efficiency; and moreover, Chinese medical therapies did not yield any side-effect.

We have seen some colleagues in Chinese medicine in Europe and in China who are a little bit shy to say something about astrology because they have known already that this for the Westerners is nonsense, but this is a wrong behaviour. You should not follow the rules of the Westerners. You know the presupposition of the doctrine of five periods and six qi is *Tian Ren He Yi* 天人合一 or the Universe and Man Uniting and Resembling Each Other (Tian 天 is usually translated into the Heaven, but is really not the same, here we use Universe instead of Heaven), and it works, that is to say, the idea "rhythms of the universe influence rhythms of the living systems by paradigm" can be understood by the way of Chinese thinking.

And now in Vienna in my seminar I would ask at this point: "Why is the astrology, the influence of the stars so undiscussable, so unimpossible for the Westerner"? But here I answer by myself. The answer is that the Western science is thinking in the way, in the manner of action and reaction, in the manner of direct influence, of cause and outcome and so on. Therefore if somebody of you – we don't believe that this will be the case – if somebody of you would say: "Yes, even the stars have influence on our lives", then you are already Westernized. The stars have no influence on our life but the performance of the stars makes understandable something which is going on in our life. This is the first try to explain this. It is very hard. Maybe here not so hard like in Vienna but it is very hard because here you must really take out all this stuff from the Western thinking and go back to old China. Keep in mind first that here already we need the concept of metaphor.

### 1.3 *QU-XIANG BI-LEI*: Circularl reasoning and phenomena

The explanation of the function of metaphor will come clearer and clearer in the next chapter of the paper. Let us now overview a little bit the Chinese science. We have discussed a lot about the *Qu-xiang Bi-Lei*. Besides of other aspects, the *Qu-xiang Bi-Lei* has two important aspects we should make understandable here:

The one is that the run of thinking is circular, is not direct, is not straight forward, but is circular. Circular thinking means that one point is explained by all the others and as soon as you go around and go to all the others in the way of knowledge you explain more and more the one point. In the Western science you try to explain by influence. This is direct way. It reduces so much. It excludes so much. In the Chinese science nothing is excluded. You go around and take all what can be related to your present question in that circular run.

The other very important point of difference to Western thinking is that for the Westerners it is always important what is remaining, what is here for all the times. For the Chinese thinking more important are the phenomena. What is going up, coming up at the moment? This is an important difference in ontology between Chinese and Western thinking. Only who is able to understand this difference understands that Western thinking must be incomparable with the Chinese science, because Western thinking is looking in Western medicine for something else than Chinese medicine.

### 1.4 Chinese Medicine: The underlining of construction against description

In difference to the descriptive Western medicine the Chinese medicine is constructive. This is always the background why from the first beginning of my activities in China at Institutes of Chinese Medicine they always liked the Constructive Realism. I was happy about it but I was also a little bit wondering why they liked it so much? Because they made this right association that construction is more similar, is closer to the way of Chinese medicine than description. We make here also a point to avoid misunderstanding. The constructivism in the Western discussion is a very manifold philosophical system, very different to philosophical schools; most of them are related to Western science.

We do not discuss here all these different ways. We just want to mention that in different to these other schools of Constructivism, the Constructive Realism is combining the constructive activities with the activities of interpreting.And this is the way of Chinese medicine: interpreting by constructing, constructing by interpretation. Now, let us go to the function of metaphor.

## 2. The function of metaphor in the structure of Chinese medicine

Metaphor is an important field of study shared in rhetoric, linguistics and philosophy. Metaphor originally refers to a rhetorical skill, a figure of speech, but is given a much more extensive meaning by logic pragmatics, referring to phenomena of meaning transfer of language in the course of expression and exchange.[1]

Metaphor is also a basic cognitive activity. Metaphor in language use is the medium as well as the result of metaphoric cognitive activities of human beings. Metaphor is an indispensable means by which human beings cognize the world.

Language by itself contains a system of metaphor. This system is closely connected with human beings' thinking system. Languages and symbols have become a complete model that a nation regards the world. Human beings have made themselves a whole. While metaphor is used, it brings back to life the image of human beings in nature and the nature of human beings as well.

If we take an example such as a simple formulation in Chinese medicine like heat in the lungs, then the Westerner will find it ridiculous or he will ask: "How can we measure it"? And at Vienna University – you know I give 14 years of seminars on Chinese medicine – I have the experience that at every seminar my students would first ask: "It must be possible somehow principally to measure the heat in this example"? And only if it is possible for them to grasp my explanation on metaphor, then they will remain in the seminar. Who cannot grasp this explanation, leave. And it is better for them if they leave.

### 2.1 Metaphor: Revealing relations

Metaphor is also in the Western world very often misunderstood. They believe that metaphor is a description by picture instead of an exact description. This is totally wrong. Metaphor is not at all a description. Let us look to a simple example from the poetical level. In the poetical language you can find such formulation like "the soldier was fighting like a lion". In this example they do not want to say that the soldier is a lion. They do not want to describe the soldier as a lion but they want to say something about the relation between the soldier and his objects, between the soldier and the enemy. The relation is described by the metaphor. Metaphor does not describe objects. Metaphor reveals relations, relations done by actions.

1 Zhou Liquan. Logic: Theory of Correct Thinking and Efficient Communication[M]. Beijing: People's Publishing House, 1994: 489.

Therefore metaphor has the function of the relation between different phenomena – let us say in this way.

Therefore heat in the lungs says nothing about the temperature in the lungs. Heat in the lungs connects the concepts of lungs – which cannot be identified with the lungs in the Western medicine – with a series of phenomena of heat, such as coughing, fever, thirsty, restlessness, constipation, dark yellow urine, red tongue with yellowish coating, fast pulse, and so on. Therefore this example means that under this condition there is heat in the lungs. You can make understandable the behaviour or the emotions or the pains or the medical dysfunctions of a person if you connect phenomena which are together somehow with heat.

We are fascinated by this idea. It is totally different from the Western science but it makes sense definitely in the details that Chinese medicine can only work if she makes clear which aspects of heat are important in explaining or understanding a disease. The detailed research must reveal which aspects of heat we can use in the circular reasonning for a specific dysfunction of the living system. Chinese medicine works well if she finds out – in respect to our example – which aspects of heat are important for a specific dysfunction of a living system. Therefore here you can see first the thinking of Chinese medicine is – if we use Chinese medicine correctly – an exact thinking, not a thinking by opinions or so.

## 2.2 Metaphorizing: An exact thinking

We definitely warn you here from one misunderstanding which is maybe in China not really strong but which can be strong in Europe. It is not the case that the difference between Western science and Chinese medicine is that Western natural science is exact and Chinese medicine is not exact. No, Chinese medicine is even more exact than the Western medicine, which we can show you by the following examples.

An example that Chinese medicine is more exact in explaining the living system is a kind of stomach disease: peptic ulcer disease. Six patients with stomach pain are all diagnosed as having peptic ulcer disease by using upper-gastrointestinal X-ray or endoscopy by means of a fiberscope. Then of course they will be given the same treatment. The physician then sends the patients to a doctor of Chinese medicine for examination. Then the six patients are diagonosed as having six different patterns of imbalances: “deficient yin affecting the stomach” (usually known as “stomach yin deficiency"), "deficient cold affecting the spleen" (usually known as "spleen yang deficiency"), "damp heat affecting the spleen", "excess cold dampness affecting the spleen & stomach", "disharmony of congealed blood in the stomach", and "disharmony of the liver invading the spleen". Then of couse they will be given 6 individualized treatments based on different patterns.[1]

Another example is the blood pressure. If we measure the blood pressure with the machine, we will be happy if it is not too high. It is too high, doctors of Western medicine will say, take the pill. They do not qualify what is the background of the blood pressure. But Chinese medicine may identify patiens with hypertension as having different patterns such as "hyperactivity of liver fire", "yin deficiency and yang hyperactivity", "pattern of phlegm turbidity", or "pattern of phlegm and blood stasis", etc., who are given individualized treatments according to different specific patterns by doctor of Chinese medicine. It is worth to note here that Chinese medical treatments may not directly lower the blood pressure, but can be used as auxillary treatments for they are effective in relieving hypertension patients' common symptoms such as headache, vertigo, insomnia, tinnitus, and so on, and in stabilizing the blood pressure, softening the blood vessels, and preventing the situation from deteriorating.

Another common example is the inflammation of the Western medicine. Inflammation is a pathological condition in Western medicine, manifesting in local redness, swelling, pain, ulcer and dysfunction as well as fever of different degrees, leukocytosis, fatigue, poor appetite, and so on, which is usually treated by antibiotics. While inflammation in Chinese medicine can be identified eight patterns: warm heat pattern, damp heat pattern, fire toxin pattern, deficient fire pattern (fire is caused by yin deficiency), wind cold pattern or cold dampness pattern, phlegm fluid pattern (with edema), deficient cold pattern (cold is caused by yang deficiency), stagnation of qi and blood (with pain). These patterns are not fixed, may vary according to the progression or retrogression of the disease. But anyway, doctor of Chinese medicine prescribes different formulas according to different patterns, i.e. identifying patterns and applying proper treatments. It is really amazing for Chinese medicine does not yield drug resistance like

---

1 Kaptchuk, Ted J. Chinese Medicine: The Web That Has No Weaver [M]. Revised ed. London: Rider, 2000: 4-6

antibiotics do, and it works even when the agent(s) of disease cannot be identified.

The above examples show that Chinese medicine is even more exact than Western natural science in the clinical practice. Besides, *Tiao Ji Tu* 太极图 or Yin-Yang Diagram, one of the vital philosophical foundations of Chinese medicine is also more exact than one of the vital philosophical foundations of Western science – Dichotomy.

As you know, a dichotomy is any splitting of a whole into exactly two non-overlapping parts. In other words, it is a bipartition of elements which are mutually exclusive, nothing can belong simultaneously to both parts, and everything must belong to one part or the other. Dichotomy is directly applied in mathematics, philosophy or linguistics. For example, if there is a concept A, and it is split into parts B and not-B, then the parts form a dichotomy: they are mutually exclusive, since no part of B is contained in not-B and vice-versa, and they are jointly exhaustive, since they cover all of A, and together again give A.[1] In the anthropologic field of theology and in philosophy as well as in the Western medicine, dichotomy is the belief that humans consist of a soul or mind and a body, which is a vital cultural presupposition of the Western medicine. Western medicine focuses on studying the human body from a system to separate organs, to cells, to genes, and so on, therefore it is good at treating body diseases such as the development of surgery, but as regards to psychosomatic diseases it cannot achieve satisfactory therapeutic effects.

*Tiao Ji Tu* 太极图 or Yin-Yang Diagram shows that in Chinese thinking everything in the universe has two facets: one yin aspect and one yang aspect; yin contains the seed of yang, and vice versa; yin and yang create, counterbalance (or wax and wane), transform into each other. Dichotomy is like “1”, while *Tiao Ji Tu* 太极图 or Yin-Yang Diagram is like “S”, much more complicated than dichotomy, therefore more exact and fitting to the living system. You know Chinese medicine is constructed under the guideline of *Tian Ren He Yi*, and the object of Chinese medicine is human being, composed the body, mind and other aspects. Chinese medicine can usually achieve desired therapeutic effects in treating psychosomatic diseases.

---

1 http://en.wikipedia.org/wiki/Dichotomy

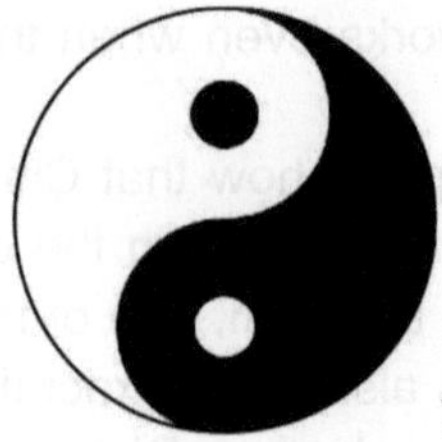

*Tai Ji Tu* 太极图

You know now why Chinese Medicine is more exact than Western science and it is clear that we cannot explain this with the traditional Philosophy of Science. We must have another Philosophy of Science which reveals the background, the conditions and preconditions, the presuppositions of the Western science. And that is what I have developed in the last twenty years – the Constructive Realism.

We could make this much clearer by another example. For the Western medicine the body is a cooperation of atoms, electrons and so on. For the Chinese medicine the living system is like a text, like a composition of words and every word can be understood by the other words. And you cannot understand one word fully if you don't know all the other words. Now you can see the source of the exactness of Chinese medicine. The text offers so much on knowledge, on information, much more than the stabilized objects of the Western medicine.

In the Western medicine – referring to our example – the lungs are an object which is clearly defined by its place and its functions and there are some diseases possible which are clearly defined and all other things are uninteresting. For example, in Chinese medicine, constipation caused by the heat in the lungs can be effectively relieved by the therapeutic methods of clearing the heat in the lungs; but in Western medicine, constipation is not associated with and treated through treating the lungs. This is reducing so much the possible information that a living system can offer. In a difficult text in Philosophy or Poetry you can understand a word only if you understand the full text. You must go always around. You cannot read at the beginning the full text, you must read word by word and then you must find out what is the meaning of the word of this text.

We think this is fascinating. This is the motivation for us to study this science because it is incredible fascinating – what can be done in interpreting a text.

3. The difference between explaining and understanding in respect to Chinese medicine

Now we explain or make you aware about an important principal difference between Western science and Chinese medicine: the difference between explaining and understanding.

Simply we could say explaining is the way of Western science, understanding the way of Chinese medicine. Explaining means we are using rules to make clear something. We give you a simple example. Maybe some of you have already thought or even say it maybe: "My parents do not understand me!" But the parents usually are explaining your behaviour – if it is strange for them – by the rules of pedagogics or by the rules of psychology. But even if somebody is explained by these rules, and we can say a girl or a boy with 14 or 15 years ago will behave in this way, and then we can explain, if she or he is destroying the furniture at home, we can say this is connected with the rules of human development. This is explaining but this girl or this boy will say: "They don't understand me".

In difference to this we should ask here what it is meant by "understanding". Sometimes people are connecting understanding with explaining. We can understand something if somebody has explained it but this is not what we mean.

We give you a simple example: For instance, if you don't understand the mathematics, then a good teacher explains the rules of mathematics. And then you say, "Now I can understand the mathematics". This means you can apply the adequate rules. Sometimes understanding is good in the way of explaining. For instance we do not know how to use these things. If somebody explains, we say, now we have understood but in this case we have only learned to apply rules, nothing else.

Applying rules is totally strange for Chinese medicine. This is one argument why Western pharmacology does not need the herbal theory of Chinese medicine – because Chinese medicine is a totally different structure, and many other arguments which we have discussed already. Understanding in this sense needs acceptance. Understanding is somehow accepting. Therefore applying the difference between Western medicine and Chinese medicine, we can say: The Western doctor explains a disease; the Chinese medical doctor makes the situation of the human being understandable for him by accepting this way. Acceptance here means that we are willing to go the circular way, the way to the different possibilities of metaphors to make understandable, to make acceptable for us the state of this living system. Acceptance here leads the way we are going in the circular reasonning. The way is depending from the living system which we should treat as a doctor.

References


[1] http://en.wikipedia.org/wiki/Dichotomy

[2] Kaptchuk, Ted J. Chinese Medicine: The Web That Has No Weaver [M]. Revised ed. London: Rider, 2000.

[3] Wallner, Friedrich. Five Lectures on the Foundations of TCM [M]. Frunkfurt am Main: Peter Lang, 2009: 27-34.

[4] Zhou Liquan. Logic: Theory of Correct Thinking and Efficient Communication[M]. Beijing: People's Publishing House, 1994: 489.

Dingfang Cai

# Hyperactivity Causing Disorders & Proper Restriction Ensuring Harmony: the Most Powerful Medicine in Human Body

When I just started to learn medicine, Mr.Xiao Fengzhang taught me with a book entitled *Yu Yi Cao* 寓意草.[1] I admired very much Mr.Yu Xichang's correct and profound insight that "Medicine is beyond any medical techniques" and that "The mechanism of disease should be mulled over and figured out before treatment". However, as regards to the quotation that "the most powerful medicine resides in the human body" from a case record named “Jin Daobin’s True Yang Deserting from the Upper” in that book, I had not truly understood although I had been mulling over it again and again until I read *Plain Questions* again 30 years later.

Time flies in a blink of eyes, and I have already spent thirty years studying medicine. In the late autumn of 2004, I read *Plain Questions* once more. I suddenly realized that the idea of “Hyperactivity Causing Disorders & Proper Restriction Ensuring Harmony” is so fabulous when I came across “Hyperactivity will do harm, so restriction is necessary. Restriction ensures generation and transformation.”, a quotation from the chapter of “Comprehensive Discourse on the Subtle Significance of the Six Atmospheric Influences” (Liu Wei Zhi Da Lun, 六微旨大论). Isn't Restriction the most powerful medicine in the human body? Kang means hyperactivity, excess; Hai means to harm; Cheng means to restrict, and Zhi is the outcome of restriction – harmonious state.

Hyperactivity is the basic mechanism of diseases, leading to Hai, i.e. harm; Cheng is the method of restriction, leading to Zhi, i.e. Harmony. Medicine is what defeats diseases, contains not only herbs and minerals,

1 *Yu Yi Cao* 寓意草: a famous book of case recods by Yu Chang 喻昌 in 1643. The over 60 cases in the book are typically selected, completely recorded, and precisely and appropriately analyzed, and therefore is quite influential and of guiding significance to learn, study and practice Chinese medicine for the later generations.

but also psychotherapy, dietary therapy, *Dao Yin*[1], and other physical exercises. Restriction is the medicine. I believe that as the chief of the heaven and the earth, the universe must have its subtle profound mechanism to create the myriad of beings and achieve prosperity; and as the carrier of life, the human body must have its profound rational principle to command the *zang fu* organs and achieve harmony. And what exactly is the profound rational principle? The answer is "Hyperactivity Causing Disorders & Proper Restriction Ensuring Harmony". Hereafter is my interpretation.

### 1. Interpretation with *Taiji*[2] and Yin-Yang

*Taiji* is the beginning of myriad of beings in the universe. Long before, the universe was shapeless, endless and hollow, which was in a state of *Wu Ji* (without Ultimate). Then qi started to move, which was known as state of *Tai Ji* (Supreme Ultimate); and then movement of qi created Yin-Yang and all of the other things, which existed together in a total mixture. The movement of *Taiji* results in separation of Yin-Yang, so Yin-Yang is *Taiji*; the harmony of Yin-Yang results in the formation of *Taiji*, so *Taiji* is Yin-yang.

Since the universe has the sun, the moon, the five phases and six climates, the human body has Yin-Yang, five viscera and six meridians. Therefore, the universe and man resemble each other, and the human body mirrors the universe. "As Heaven's movement is ever vigorous, a gentleman should ceaselessly strive along for his self-perfection; As Earth's condition is receptive devotion, a gentleman should hold the outer world with his broad mind".[3] The mechanism of the universe lies in movement and stillness. The heaven starts with movement, which leads to generation; while the earth starts with stillness, which leads to transformation.

1 *Dao Yin*, or conducting exercise 导引: an ancient Chinese physical exercise associated with respiratory movement and self-massage performed by conducting the mind and qi, used for health preservation and disease prevention and treatment.

2 *Taiji* or the Supreme Ultimate: the Absolute in ancient Chinese cosmology, presented as the primary source of all created things, i.e. *qi*.

3 This is a famous quotation on Trigram Qian 乾 and Trigram Kun 坤 respectively from *The Book of Changes*.

If the movement is in excess, the stillness restricts it; if Yang is in hyperactivity, Yin restricts it. Thus interaction of the movement and stillness, and waning and waxing between Yin and Yang result in harmony of everything in the universe. *The Book of Changes* states that the interaction of the heaven qi and the earth qi creates all things in the universe. It is really indeed the case! Creation of all of the beings is the outcome of harmonious interaction between movement and stillness. Without movement there is no change; while without stillness there is no transformation. Changes and transformations will stop if without movement and stillness; while upbearing, downbearing, entering and existing will terminate if without change and transformation. Without entering and exiting of qi, then the life will dim; without upbearing and downbearing of qi, the body's functional activities will stop.

The lungs reside in the upper part of the body, commanding qi of the whole body; while the kidneys reside in the lower part of the body, governing water of the whole body. Water transforms into qi, and qi condenses into water, which indicates that the lungs (metal) and the kidneys (water) moisten and benefit each other. The lungs govern the exiting of qi, while the kidneys dominate the entering of qi (or the receiving of qi), which makes qi movement in a balanced state.

The liver is a tough viscus, governing free coursing; while the lungs are a delicate viscus, commanding purifying, cleansing, and descending. The liver qi upbears from the left while the lung qi downbears from the right, showing a balanced qi movement between upbearing and downbearing, entering and exiting, which ensures the normal life activities. Therefore, there would be no birth, growth, transformation, harvest, and storage in the nature if without movement and stillness; and there would be no birth, growth, maturity, decline and death in man if without movement and stillness.

*Taiji*, the same as Yin-Yang, is the way of heaven and earth, the principle governing myriad of beings, the father and mother to all the changes and transformations, the root and beginning of generating and killing. However, everything exists on its counterpart. Everything has its father and mother, just like mayfly has the male and the female; everything has *Taiji*, just like a particle has the positive and the negative. Both movement and stillness should be changed in a proper range. If the movement is in excess, it's called hyperactivity; if the stillness is in excess, it's also called hypoactivity. Neither hyperactivity nor hypoactivity is good. Excess without restriction is hyperactivity, which is harmful for it leads to natural disasters in the nature or social problems in the society or diseases in man. Thus, everything in the universe needs to be restrained. Restriction in the nature makes the four seasons alternate in a gentle way; restriction in the society makes it full of virtue behaviors; restriction between the heart (fire) and the kidneys (water) makes the whole body in a harmonious state for heart fire downbears to warm up kidney water and kidney water upbears to restrain heart fire. Fire is hot in nature, so without water it will cause yin exhaustion and burn out everything; water is cold in nature, so without fire it will cause yang exhaustion and perish everything. Restriction ensures harmony. The nature and the society will then be in a perfect order when balanced. Hyperactivity will do harm and harm will cause suffering. That is the time to use restriction as a cure, not only for the human body, but also for the whole universe. Kidney water is the true water which restricts fire, and heart fire is the true fire which restricts water. When the genuine yang in the kidneys upbears naturally, qi will engender like the sunrise in the coldest dawn; when the genuine yin in the heart downbears naturally, qi will engender like the dusk in the hottest day. So no matter how many principles exist in between yin and yang, harmony is the essence. *Lao Tzu* states that "Tao produces one, one produces two. The two produce three and the three produce all things. All things in the universe carry yin and embrace yang, where the central qi makes them in harmony"[1]. So if one keeps yin even and yang firm, one's spirit will be sound. The waning and waxing between yin and yang is the way of generation and transformation; the counterbalance between yin and yang is the mechanism of "restriction ensuring harmony". So the ways of yin and yang is indeed the most powerful medicine in the human body and the universe. How the herbal medicine could be compared with! You see how profound and true Mr. Yu Xichang's formulations are!

2. Interpretation with the Five Phases

The five phases refer to wood, fire, earth, metal and water. Wood is the bending and straightening and governs dispersing, corresponding to the

---

1 From the Chapter 42 of *Lao Tzu*.

east and the green-blue dragon, and dominating the spring wind; the liver (wood) governs free coursing, opens into the eyes, and rules the sinews. Fire is the flaming upwards and governs warming, corresponding to the south and the red bird, and dominating the summer heat; the heart (fire) governs the spirit, opens into the tongue, and rules the vessels. Earth is the sowing and reaping and governs sweltering, corresponding to the center and the Saturn[1], and dominating the late summer dampness; the spleen (earth) governs movement and transformation, opens into the mouth, and rules the flesh. Metal is the working of change and governs astringing, corresponding to the west and the Venus[2], dominating the autumn dryness; the lungs (metal) govern respiration, open into the nose, and rule the surface of the body. Water is the moistening and downward flowing and governs moistening, corresponding to the north and the black tortoise, and dominating the winter coldness; the kidneys govern the essence and water metabolism, open into the ears, and rule the bones.

I have heard that the properties of the five phases are used for categorization, while their functions lie in the engendering and restricting relationship among them. Therefore, engendering and restricting imply in the categorization according to the five phases. Water engenders wood, wood engenders fire, fire engenders earth, earth engenders metal and metal engenders water. Water restricts fire, fire restricts metal, metal restricts wood, wood restricts earth and earth restricts water. All of the beings in the universe can be categorized according to the five phases, and thus engendering and restricting among them happen all the time. The engendering and restricting form an endless and ceaseless cycle, which is the way of the heaven and the earth.

As for the human beings, if engendering and restricting among the five phases are in the right order and to a proper degree, the viscera can function well by themselves and cooperate well with each other, qi and blood can flow smoothly inside the vessels, mind and spirit are lucid, the body metabolism is normal, the physique is strong, and hence a long life can be expected. The normal engendering and restricting among the five

---

1 The Saturn is "Earth Star 土星" in Chinese for its color was yellow in ancient Chinese eyes and yellow is the color of Earth phase.

2 The Venus is "Metal Star 金星" or "Great White 太白" in Chinese for it was big and bright in ancient Chinese eyes and white is the color of Metal Phase.

phases in the body not only can control disease with mind, but also can prevent disease from occurring before its onset. The universe was in a mess without any rules and regulations before the five phases came out; while all things started to function in a rational way after the five phases came out, and the five phases are just like a wise emperor who governed the country properly and put everything into order.[1] Ancient Chinese people, however, merged this philosophical thought into medicine and developed it very well ever since.

All the people know that engendering is good, but few understand that over-engendering leads to excess, which is bad. For example, when water is in excess and it will be flooding, and the kidneys will be affected; when fire is in excess and it will be raging, and the heart will be affected; when wood is in excess and it will be breaking out, and the liver will be affected; when metal is in excess and it will be killing, and the lungs will be affected; when earth is in excess and it will be blocking, and the spleen will be affected. So there must be a powerful medicine inside to control them, and which is exactly the mechanism of restriction. See, when water is in excess, fire will come to restrict it; and vice versa; when metal is in excess, fire will come to restrict it; when wood is in excess, metal will come to restrict it; when earth is in excess, wood will come to restrict it. Restricting leads to harmony, and harmony ensures normal generation and transformation. That is why restricting works in the body all the time! That is why restriction is the most powerful medicine in the body!

However, hypoactive restricting can be overcome by engendering. See, dim fire can be flaming again if getting engendered by wood; dull metal can be sharp again if getting engendered by earth; depressive wood can be free and smooth again if getting engendered by water; barren earth can be fertile again if getting engendered by fire; insufficient water can be used to irrigate again if getting engendered by metal. That is the way of engendering, which is also supplementary and complementary to restricting. Engendering results in restricting, and restricting leads to generation and transformation. Therefore engendering works in the body every minute and second.

---

1 The formulation here means that the theory of five phases is a rational doctrine to interprete the working of the universe.

Kidney is the foundation of prenatal existence and the spleen is the foundation of postnatal existence, and therefore they interact with each other to govern the original qi, which consists of the postnatal qi and the prenatal qi. The postnatal qi makes life prosperous after gaining the prenatal qi; and the prenatal qi starts endless transformations after gaining the postnatal qi. Liver is yin in nature but prefers free coursing, while spleen is still but functions to move and transform. Liver's free coursing promotes movement and transformation of water and grain, and spleen's function of movement and transformation nourishes the liver's free coursing; they benefit each other, and thus make life prosperous. Heart commands blood of the whole body and lungs command qi of the whole body, and they both reside in the upper energizer[1] and both dominate the flow of qi and blood. The respiration is in harmony if the lungs get the nourishment from the heart blood, and the blood flows smoothly if the heart gets the pushing force from the lung qi. Therefore, qi is the commander of blood and blood flows along with qi; while blood is the mother of qi and qi is calm when it attaches blood. Lung qi disperses, purifies and downbears water fluids; spleen qi functions to move and transform water fluids. *Huang Di's Inner Classic* states that: "Fluids taken in enter the stomach. Here, they are churned and their essential qi is strained off. This is then carried to the spleen and further distributed by spleen qi. It passes up to the lungs which regulate the waterways down to the bladder. Thus water essence is distributed to the four parts, (by) passing through the five channels."[2] Isn't engendering another powerful medicine in the body? In the mechanism of the created universe, engendering is of the same significance as restricting for without any one of them the balance will be interrupted, which will

---

1 The upper energizer refers to Shang Jiao 上焦. Energizer is a standard translation for Jiao 焦, which is approved by World Health Organization, such as Triple Energizer for San Jiao 三焦. Actually, Burner is more popular in the English literature on Chinese medicine published in the West. But actually both translations are misleading. Pinyin transliteration is the best but far away from well-known, so the standard translation "Energizer" is adopted here to avoid misunderstanding. See LAN Fengli. A Corpus-Based Study on Cultural Connotations and Translation of Fundamental Concepts in Classical Chinese Texts (Post-Doctoral Report). Shanghai: Shanghai Jiao Tong University, 2008.

2 From the Chapter of "Further Discourse on Vessels" or Jing Mai Bie Lun 经脉别论 of *Plain Questions* or Su Wen 素问.

definitely lead to excess and harm. So without restricting there will be no engendering. And thus, restriction is the most powerful medicine in the human body.

Please allow me to give you some further interpretation. People possess the five phases, and grow along with the wind qi. The wind qi can also harm the beings although it usually promotes their growth, which is just like the water can carry the boat on and also can capsize it. After disease arises, a herbal prescription is given to attack, to supplement, to clear, to disperse, to cause sweating, or to precipitate based on pattern identification. Why can herbal medicine cure disease? The reason is that the mechanism of "Hyperactivity Causing Disorders & Proper Restriction Ensuring Harmony" also lies in the disease itself, and the function of herbal medicine is to restore its role of restriction so as to rectify a deviation and correct an error as well as to support the healthy qi and dispel pathogenic influences, thus to cure the disease. If restriction does not function, even the most distinguished doctors such as Bian Que can do nothing to bring the life back. And this is another interpretation of "Hyperactivity Causing Disorders & Proper Restriction Ensuring Harmony", "the most powerful medicine in the human body". Alas! The manifestations of the changing process of disease are visible and can be known, while the mechanism of the inner balance is invisible and cannot be predicted. The invisible one is infinite and hard to predict while the visible one is easy to observe. Thus, I have learned that being a doctor, the mechanism of "Hyperactivity Causing Disorders & Proper Restriction Ensuring Harmony" is essential and we must bear it in mind. Reading medical classical texts and doing medical practice is just like facing floating clouds and watching an abyss. The abyss is limpid, and its depth can be easily estimated; the clouds are randomly floating, so their margins are far away from known when facing them. Visible objects are like the observable abyss, while the way of changing is like unpredictable clouds. When I face a patient, a sense of invisibility comes to me. I would like to devote myself to the profound and subtle way of practicing Chinese medicine.

I am just like a summer worm who talks about the ice, and never know how great the universe is. What I have discussed here is shallow and incomplete. And so I sincerely welcome all kinds of critical suggestions or positive comments from you. [1]

1 Translator's note: The formulation here is the author's self-deprecating remarks made as a gesture of politeness. Actually, the author is a professor and MD supervisor of Fudan University, and highly qualified in classical Chinese medicine and Western medicine.

**Badie, Kambi** received all his degrees from Tokyo Institute of Technology, Japan, majoring in pattern recognition. Within the past years, he has been actively involved in doing research in a variety of issues, such as machine learning, cognitive modeling, knowledge processing & creation in general, and analogical knowledge processing, experience modeling and modeling interpretation process in particular, with emphasis on generating new ideas, techniques and contents as well. His familiarity with Constructive Realism and its main strategy (strangification) gave him an opportunity to investigate his desired topics from the viewpoint of this epistemological movement. Within this context he has developed a number of approaches using strangification as a core strategy for analogical reasoning as well as interpretation processes. Out of these approaches, "interpretative approach to analogical reasoning", as well as "viewpoint oriented manipulation of concepts" are particularly mentionable as novel approaches to creative idea generation. Dr. Badie is an ex-director of IT Research Faculty in Iran Telecom Research Center and at present an advisor to the center's director for IT affairs. Email: k_badie@itrc.ac.ir

**Cai, Dingfang**, born in 8th November, 1956 in Shanghai, China; Cai obtained PhD from Nanjing Traditional Chinese Medicine University in 1988, then worked as a visiting scholar in the Medical Center of the University of Tokushima, Japan from July 1990 to July 1991, and as a Post-PhD in Toyama Medical and Pharmaceutical University from September 1994 to September 1995. Cai built the foundation of a strong TCM & Integrative medicine research with Academician Shen Ziyin, then he accomplished a training course aimed specifically at the solid and broad basic theory, as well as the deep and systemic expertise. He is expert in the TCM & Integrative medicine therapy and research in Neurology, and active in the front line of medication, teaching and research. His achievements got favorable comments from others of the same occupation. He assumed the responsibility of tackling key problems in China – Japan cooperation, National Key Technologies R&D Programs, National Natural Science Foundation of China (NSFC), as well as many other projects from Ministry of Public

Health, Education, and the State Administration of Traditional Chinese Medicine. Currently Chief director of Traditional Chinese Medicine & Integrative Medicine Department of Zhongshan Hospital, Medical Center, Fudan University; Professor; Doctoral Advisor; Associate Director of Institute of Integrated Traditional and Western Medicine, Fudan University; Director of Integrative Neurological Research Office of Institute of Integrative Medicine, Fudan University; Contact of Key Subject of Integrative Medicine, Fudan University.

**Duan, Yishan**, Shanghai University of Traditional Chinese Medicine, born on July 16th 1940 in Shanghai, graduated from the major of Chinese Language and Literature of Fudan University in July 1965. Currently life-tenure professor, PhD supervisor at Shanghai University of Traditional Chinese Medicine. Has been the chief compiler of the fifth, the sixth and the seventh editions of *Ancient Medical Chinese* (Yi Gu Wen), the national textbook for higher education of Chinese medicine in China. Other works include *Rhetoric of Ancient Chinese Medical Language*, *Methods to Identify Meanings of Words in Ancient Chinese Medical Texts*, *Practical Ancient Medical Chinese*, *New Compilation of Ancient Medical Chinese*, *Selected Rare Ancient Hand Copies on Chinese Medicine*, etc. Has published over 100 papers. Has won Excellent Teacher Award of Baogang Steel Education Fund and Shanghai Prize for Advancement of Science and Technology. His name has been included into the *List of World-Famous Persons* by International Biographical Centre (IBC, Cambridge, England) Scientific Emphases: Ancient Medical Chinese; History, Literature and Culture of Chinese Medicine; Language of Chinese Medicine.

**Gao, Junpeng**, born in 1979, studied Integrative Medicine and Chinese Medicine (Bachelor and Master in Chinese Medicine at Shanghai University of TCM, Doctor of Integrative Chinese Medicine at Fudan University). Currently Attending Physician of the Department of Integrative Medicine & Traditional Chinese Medicine, Zhongshan Hospital, Fudan University; Quality Assurance for Clinical Research Professionals of Shanghai Clinical Research Center; Secretary and Member of Neurological Division of Shanghai Association of Chinese Medicine; Member of Shanghai Academy of Integrative Medicine Youth Committee. Has published over 20 papers in high-level refereed academic journals. Scientific Emphases: Clinical and basic research in treating Neurological, psychiatrical diseases with integrated Chinese-Western therapy.

**Lan, Fengli**, Shanghai University of Traditional Chinese Medicine, born in 1972, studied Medicine, esp. Chinese Medicine (Bachelor in Medicine in 1995 at Hebei Medical University, Master in Medicine in 1998 and PhD in Discipline of Medicine in 2005 at Shanghai University of Traditional Chinese Medicine) English Language and Literature (B.A. in 2003 at Shanghai International Studies University), and Applied Linguistics (Post-Doctoral Researcher in Applied Linguistics in 2008 at Shanghai Jiao Tong University). Currently associate professor for applied linguistics at Shanghai University of TCM since January 2008. She has published eight books in China and over 30 papers in high-level refereed academic journals. Selected Publications: Treatment of Anovulatory Menstruation with Therapy of Artificial Menstrual Cycle Achieved Through Selection of Acupoints (2002); The Influence of Translator Subjectivities on English Translation of *Huang Di Nei Jing Su Wen* (2005); Influence of *Huangdi's Inner Classic* on *The Origin of Chinese Characters* (2006); The Origin of Yin-Yang as Chinese Medical Terms and Their Translation (2007); Philosophical Reflections on Standardization of English Chinese Medical Terminology (2010); Constructive Realism and Its Enlightenments for Researching Chinese Medicine (2010); etc. Scientific Emphases (in the last two decades): Foundations, Acupuncture, Gynecology, History and Literature of Chinese Medicine; Trans-cultural and Translation Studies of Chinese Medicine; Applied Linguistics; English Language and Literature; and Philosophy of Science.

**Litscher, Gerhard**, born in 1958 in Graz, Austria. Head of the Research Unit of Biomedical Engineering in Anesthesia and Intensive Care Medicine and of the TCM Research Center Graz at the Medical University of Graz, Doctor of technical and Doctor of medical sciences, several research stays and international lectures, about 500 scientific publications, partly on basic acupuncture research, author and/or editor of eleven books, currently editor-in-chief and/or member of the editorial board of 20 international scientific journals. http://tcm-graz.at, http://litscher.info

**Mahmoudi, Maryam Tayefeh** is a Ph.D candidate at department of machine intelligence in the University of Tehran. Within the past years, she has been involved in a variety of research works at IT Research Faculty of Iran Telecom Research Center working on issues like automatic content generation/creation as well as conceptualization of IT research projects. She has been interested in strangification as a helpful strategy for creating knowledge in general and generating contents in particular. She is a co-author of the book entitled "Strangification: A New Paradigm in Knowledge Processing & Creation" and also the co-author of a number of research papers (together with Dr.Badie) with regard to applications of strangification to automated reasoning. At present she is a researcher at Knowledge Engineering & Intelligent Systems Group in IT Research Faculty of Iran Telecom Research Center, and in the meantime a lecturer of computer engineering subjects in the University of Tehran. Email: Mahmodi @itrc.ac.ir

**Qin, Jianguo**, MD & PHD, Associate Professor, Dongfang hospital, Beijing university of Chinese Medicine. Education: Bachelor in1994, Department of Chinese Traditional medicine, Hebei Medical University. Doctor of Medicine and Philosophy in 2005, Beijing University of Chinese Medicine. Post-doctor in 2009, Center of Biomolecular Medicine and Pharmacology, Department of Vascular Biology and Thrombosis Research, Medical University of Vienna. Now research Chinese traditional medicine combined with western medicine to prevent and treat renal fibrosis rat and the kidney protection mechanism of JYTMF on Hypertension nephrosclerosis. Awards: 2008: the project Supported by Doctoral Fund of Ministry of Education of China "Effect of reversing vascular remodeling in hypertension nephrosclerosis and regulation on adrenomedullin signal transduction pathway by treatment with Pinggantongluo method" 2006: Partner in the project of National natural science foundation "the research of the mechanism of alterations in signaling pathway during left ventricular remodeling in hypertension by treatment with improving blood and calming heart methods". Publications: 10 books and more than 20 articles about Chinese Medicine.

**Riegel, Andrea-Mercedes**, independent scholar, was born in 1957. She studied Applied Linguistics and French and Spanish Languages in Heidelberg (diploma 1983). She took up studies in Chinese Language, Literature and Philosophy in 1984 and lived in Taiwan between 1989 and 1991 where she studied Chinese Medicine at a private high school. Back in Germany she finished her studies in Heidelberg and took up her doctoral studies in Munich (Doctoral thesis in philosophy accomplished in 1999). At the same time she intensified her studies in integrative and natural medicine in Mannheim. Since 1999 she works as a practitioner of Chinese medicine in Heidelberg and meanwhile accomplished a second doctoral dissertation in medical sciences (University of Witten-Herdecke). She published nine books and numerous articles about acupuncture and TCM treatment of different health problems and chronic diseases. Selected publications: Fibromyalgia – questions and answers from the point of view of Chinese Medicine (2001), The female organism in Chinese medicine – menstrual disorders treated with acupuncture (2001, in cooperation with Zou Hua), Diabetes and TCM – TCM as adjunct treatment of diabetes mellitus (2004), Ling Zhen – the spiritual aspects of acupuncture (2008), The Kidney *shen*, concepts of Classical Chinese medicine seen from the point of view of western medicine (2009), *Bianzheng lunzhi* – Chinese differential diagnosis of symptoms and diseases (2010), Trigeminal neuralgia treated with acupuncture (article 2010), TCM and the *Yijing* (2004, The origin of the TCM theories in the *Yijng* (2005, 4 parts), TCM and the *Yijing* tradition and modernity. Scientific emphasis: foundations of Chinese medicine, the *Yijing*, treatment of chronic diseases with TCM, interpretation of Chinese medical terms in western medicine, integration of Chinese and western medicine, translation of classical Chinese medical texts into German language

**Simon, Jeremy R.** studied medicine (MD 1994) and philosophy (PhD 2006) at NYU. He is now an emergency physician and philosopher of medicine at Columbia University, where he holds appointments in the Department of Medicine and the Center for Bioethics. His work covers both medical ethics as well as the ontology of medicine and has appeared in leading journals in philosophy and medicine.

**Tani, Toru** was born in 1954 in Ichinomiya, Japan. The main focus of his research is phenomenology and the phenomenological movement. He began his studies in philosophy at Keio University in Tokyo and was awarded a Ph.D. in philosophy at Tohoku University in Sendai. He has been teaching philosophy at various colleges and university since 1986, and since 2003, has been a professor of philosophy at Ritsumeikan University in Kyoto. Following the publication of his main work, *Ishiki no shizen* (The Physis of Consciousness), he has been developing new ways for phenomenological thinking, mainly from the aspect of intercultural phenomenology. He is currently head of the Research Center for Intercultural Phenomenology in Kyoto, established in 2009.

**Wallner, Fritz G.** is born in 1945 in Weiten, Austria. He studied a couple of disciplines (philosophy, psychology, German and classical literatures, education); after some years as a high school teacher, lecturer at the Department of Theoretical Physics and university docent (Senior lecturer); in 1987 he became Professor for Philosophy and Philosophy of Science at Vienna University. During 1985-95 development of a new philosophy of science, Constructive Realism, that makes the manifold of scientific approaches understandable in their dependence on different cultures; since 1990 intensive work on the argumentative structure of TCM; lectures in 60 countries, TCM-Teaching in Vienna University since 1994; 200 essays and 14 books, translated in 14 languages.

**Zou**, **Hua,** Dr. med., born in China in 1957, studied medicine and specialized in acupuncture. She is a member of the National Federation of Acupuncture in China. In 1992 she settled in Germany and took her doctoral degree (1997) in medicine at Heidelberg University. From 1995-2003 she conducted several research projects on acupuncture and allergies during which she developed diagnostic methods and acupuncture therapies to treat allergy-related respiratory diseases, asthma, and rhinitis. In 2005 she set up her practice for Chinese Medicine where she provides training for Medical Doctors and patients interested in Chinese Medicine. As Dr. Zou has a profound knowledge of Western and Chinese Medicine she noticed that each system has some gaps while treating patients suffering from diverse disorders. This led her to establish the Academy for Integrative Medicine in 2008 which merges the best methods of the existing medical systems, closes existing gabs, and thus comes up with a new, enhanced system. The ultimate goal is to develop preventative medicine which is based on new diagnostic methods that are easily understood and applied and yield results within 5 seconds by just locking at the patient.

**Culture and Knowledge**

Edited by Friedrich G. Wallner

Vol. 1 Friedrich G. Wallner: Structure and Relativity. 2005.

Vol. 2 Kurt Greiner: Therapie der Wissenschaft. Eine Einführung in die Methodik des Konstruktiven Realismus. 2005.

Vol. 3 Daniël Francois Malherbe Strauss: Paradigmen in Mathematik, Physik und Biologie und ihre philosophischen Wurzeln. Ins Deutsche übertragen von Martin J. Jandl. 2005.

Vol. 4 Friedrich G. Wallner: What Practitioners of TCM Should Know. A Philosophical Introduction for Medical Doctors. With a Supplement by *Kelvin Chan*. 2006.

Vol. 5 Kurt Greiner / Friedrich G. Wallner / Martin Gostentschnig (Hrsg.): Verfremdung – Strangification. Multidisziplinäre Beispiele der Anwendung und Fruchtbarkeit einer epistemologischen Methode. 2006.

Vol. 6 Kurt Greiner: Psychoanalytik als Wissenschaft des 21. Jahrhunderts. Ein konstruktivistischer Blick auf Struktur und Reflexionspotential einer polymorphen Kontextualisations-Technik. 2007.

Vol. 7 Kambiz Badie / Maryam Tayefeh Mahmoudi: Strangification: A New Paradigm in Knowledge Processing and Creation. 2007.

Vol. 8 Friedrich G. Wallner: Systemanalyse als Wissenschaftstheorie I: Von der Sprachlichkeit zur Kulturalität. Redigiert von Florian Schmidsberger und Kurt Greiner. 2008.

Vol. 9 Friedrich G. Wallner: Five Lectures on the Foundations of Chinese Medicine. Copyedited by Florian Schmidsberger. 2009.

Vol. 10 Friedrich G. Wallner / Gertrude Kubiena / Martin J. Jandl (eds.): Understanding Traditional Chinese Medicine. Consultant: Lena Springer. 2009.

Vol. 11 Fritz G. Wallner / Florian Schmidsberger / Franz Martin Wimmer (eds.): Intercultural Philosophy. New Aspects and Methods. 2010.

Vol. 12 Friedrich G. Wallner: Systemanalyse als Wissenschaftstheorie II: Kulturalismus als Perspektive der Philosophie im 21. Jahrhundert. 2010.

Vol. 13 Friedrich G. Wallner / Fengli Lan / Martin J. Jandl (eds.): The Way of Thinking in Chinese Medicine. Theory, Methodology and Structure of Chinese Medicine. 2010.

Vol. 14 Kurt Greiner / Martin J. Jandl / Friedrich G. Wallner (eds.): Aus dem Umfeld des Konstruktiven Realismus. Studien zu Psychotherapiewissenschaft, Neurokritik und Philosophie. 2010.

Vol. 15 Martin J. Jandl: Praxeologische Funktionalontologie. Eine Theorie des Wissens als Synthese von H. Dooyeweerd und R.B. Brandon. 2010.

Vol. 16 Friedrich G. Wallner: Systemanalyse als Wissenschaftstheorie III: Das Vorhaben einer kulturorientierten Wissenschaftstheorie in der Gegenwart. 2011.

Vol. 17 Friedrich G. Wallner / Fengli Lan / Martin J. Jandl (eds.): Chinese Medicine and Intercultural Philosophy. Theory, Methodology and Structure of Chinese Medicine. 2011.

www.peterlang.de

Friedrich G. Wallner / Fengli Lan / Martin J. Jandl (eds.)

# The Way of Thinking in Chinese Medicine

## Theory, Methodology and Structure of Chinese Medicine

Frankfurt am Main, Berlin, Bern, Bruxelles, New York, Oxford, Wien, 2010.
129 pp., num. tab.
Culture and Knowledge. Edited by Friedrich G. Wallner. Vol. 13
ISBN 978-3-631-61196-8 · hardback € 27,80*

Chinese Medicine is an outstanding scientific proposition system with its own structural, methodological and theoretical prerequisites flowing into the specific practices that make Chinese Medicine popular in the Western world. However, we should be aware of the fact that Chinese Medicine is challenged in its existence because it is widely unknown. Fostering the understanding of Chinese Medicine in various aspects is, hence, the main aim of this book that gives interesting insights into the discussions on current developments in Chinese Medicine research.

*Content:* Dao, Qi, and Body/Mind-Huanglao Daoist Methodology of Nurturing Life · Globalization of TCM: Cultural Differences between TCM and Western Medicine · Applied Methodologies for Teaching, Learning, Spreading and Survival of TCM · Metaphor, *Qu Xiang Bi Lei* and Chinese Medicine · Discussion of the Basic Categories in the TCM Theoretical System · TCM Essential Conception and Methods of the Theory · Ontological Ambiguity and Methodological Circularity: *Qu Xiang Bi Lei* · Structural Parallelisms in Psychoanalysis and Traditional Chinese Medicine and Their Struggle for Scientific Acknowledgement in the Western World

Frankfurt am Main · Berlin · Bern · Bruxelles · New York · Oxford · Wien
Distribution: Verlag Peter Lang AG
Moosstr. 1, CH-2542 Pieterlen
Telefax 00 41 (0) 32 / 376 17 27

*The €-price includes German tax rate
Prices are subject to change without notice

**Homepage http://www.peterlang.de**